Silica – The Amazing

To Diane
for better health
with silica

Anaheim -87

Klaus K.

Silica
THE AMAZING GEL

An essential mineral
for radiant health,
recovery and
rejuvenation

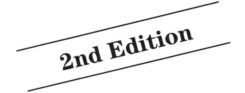

2nd Edition

Klaus Kaufmann

Foreword by Zoltan P. Rona, M.D., M.Sc.

Published by
alive books
PO Box 80055
Burnaby BC
Canada V5H 3X1

Cover Photo: Ron Crompton/Siegfried Gursche
  Crystal courtesy of The Crystalworks Gallery
  Vancouver BC
Back Cover Photo: Siegfried Gursche
Typesetting/layout: Marian MacLean
Cover Design: Bill Stockmann

First printing: January 1993
Second printing: August 1995

2nd Edition
First printing: February 1997

Canadian Cataloguing in Publication Data

Kaufmann, Klaus 1942 –
Silica : the amazing gel

Includes bibliographical references and index.
ISBN 0–920470–32–7 (bound). —ISBN 0–920470–30–0 (pbk.)

1. Silica gel—Therapeutic use. 2. Health.
I. Title. II. Author.
TX553.S5K38 1992   612.3'924   C93–091024–9

Printed and bound in Canada.

Dedicated to Gerda von Känel who
taught me faith and awakened a love
of knowledge in me

Acknowledgements

I wish to thank all who have contributed to this work. A very special thanks to the many readers of the first volume who wrote asking questions about the possible therapeutic difference between vegetal silica and mineral silica gel. Their questing comments prompted this answer. I dedicate my findings to them. I thank my publisher, Siegfried Gursche, who continuously works on creating financial and publishing opportunities.

Finally, a special thank you to my life partner Gabrielle, who looks after me with healthful drinks and meals when I am studying or staring deeply into the recesses of my computer screen, and who enthusiastically listens to my theories.

Contents

ix

Foreword
to the Second Edition

On January 1st 1997, following hoary tradition, I lifted a glass of non-sparkling, non-alcoholic, silica-rich beverage coming to me from across the great waters. I made a toast to many more great silica discoveries. The evidence before you (THIS BOOK) shows that some New Year's Resolutions are realized. Mind you, lots of new silica developments spurned me on. Thus on January 16th 1997, I received exciting news of a new medical study done in Europe that was touching on silicon. This study poignantly underlines the need for ample nutrient silica supplementation in our daily diet as acclaimed by the late Professor Carlisle.

Edith Muriel Carlisle* concentrated the research of her last years on the effect that colloidal silica supplementation can have on reversing Alzheimer's. Her preliminary findings - as she told me in 1995 – were promising. She could show that silica (or the silicon in silica!) prevents symptoms of Alzheimer's, apparently by countering the detrimental effects of aluminum.

Carlisle may not have known that in July 1993, just after the first edition of this book went to print, the British medical journal Lancet reported that researchers at the Newcastle General Hospital and at two other independent research facilities in Britain, tested the theory that silicon could react with aluminum in the human organism, thereby preventing absorption of aluminum.

---

* Edith Muriel Carlisle a professor at UCLA, and the world's foremost silica researcher, passed away in December 1995, stopping her important silica research in its tracks. According to her daughter, Wendy Carlisle, who promised to send me her mother's final papers, her research has unfortunately not been picked up or continued by any of Carlisle's past students or coworkers.

Volunteers were first given aluminum dissolved in orange juice. Then their blood was tested for aluminum. A significant amount of aluminum was found. Six weeks later, the volunteers were given aluminum and dissolved sodium silicate, a substance containing silicon. The researchers discovered that in the second challenge with aluminum no aluminum was detectable. They concluded that "since the chronic assimilation of aluminum in the brain may contribute to or accelerate the development of Alzheimer-type neuro-degenerative changes, a long-term increase in the dietary intake of silicon* could prove to be of therapeutic value."

Though the researchers did not say how those at risk of Alzheimer's disease (and that according to some research workers is quickly becoming every third person over the age of seventy) should obtain silicon, the conclusions are obvious. Sodium silicate is a scientifically purified silicon compound specifically prepared for research and not intended nor recommended as a supplement to human nutrition. Silica from silica-rich foods or supplementary silica derived from colloidal forms are the obvious choices.

In January 1997, I heard that a Dutch-Belgian medical team found, in a study done with 284 Alzheimer's patients, that Alzheimer's disease may be at least partially due to clogging of the arteries that supply the brain with oxygen and nutrients. It appears that silica may offer double protection against Alzheimer's (and possibly other forms of dementia?). Firstly, silica is intimately connected to the maintenance of the elasticity of the arterial walls (brittle arterial walls lead to clogging), and, secondly, silica challenges aluminum, which, according to Carlisle et al, is implicated in Alzheimer's.

* I prefer the term "silica" to "silicon" because elemental silicon does not occur in isolation on earth! Safe to eat colloidal silica (nutrient Silica Gel) consists of atoms of silicon (Si) bound to oxygen (O) in silica (SiO_2). Small enough particles of silica dissolved in hydrogen/oxygen (H_2O) render silica "colloidal."

Former President Reagan is nowadays languishing from symptoms of Alzheimer's. Nancy is, according to a friend of the family, a vet, who treats racehorses including the Reagan's horse, considering putting him on a nutrient silica regimen. This veterinarian telephoned me in October 1996, informing me that he followed the advice in the first edition of this book and that his medical team is achieving amazing results by putting racehorses on nutrient colloidal Silica Gel. "An amazing gel," he affirms, and continues, "I will talk to the Reagan's. Expect a phone call."

Then, in November 1996 I found out about a most exciting, new and totally natural source of a colloidal silica supplement. It comes as a delicious, pure, natural water with a silica content of 81 mg/l. This high silica content in a newly discovered natural drinking water is identical to the Dunaris spring, that I reported on in *Silica – The Forgotten Nutrient* in the chapter "A World Without Cancer." I immediately saw a possibility for a world-class Spa. I just had to go to Fiji on a journey of discovery. Chapter Four details how I found a sure prescription for natural healing with no medical doctor required!

In his hilarious "Dead Doctors Don't Lie" seminar, Joel D. Wallach, BS, DVM, ND, himself no medical doctor, succinctly informs listeners that while the average person nowadays reaches the age of 80, medical doctors on average die at age 58! Then he reminds us that the absolute span for a human's life is 140. Let's see, that is seven times the rate of physical maturity - or about 120 to 140 years - yes, he is right on for humans. More amazingly, Wallach, by the way another veterinarian (why are they seemingly ahead of MD's in medical know-how?), suggests that we could all reach 140 in good health provided only that we follow this trinity of advice:

1) we stay away from avoidable stupidities such as getting killed in a car accident.

2) we stay away from hospitals where most people die and from medical doctors, who by dying at 58 on average obviously don't know much about longevity.

3) *we continuously supply our bodies with vital colloidal minerals.*

Am I not right on the mark when I proclaim in Chapter Two: Heaven is a Colloidal? Colloidal supplements are the supplements of choice in Germany for many years!

Another reason for my New Year's toast in 1997 comes from Germany. In a loving return to my roots, I wrote this very book you are reading in my mother tongue, German. The work was published in January 1997 by the leading publisher in Germany, and, even as I am writing this, *Silicium – Heilung durch Ursubstanz* is being read for the first time in German-speaking lands. Reviewers there posed the question whether the book may not be "direction giving for therapy in the 21st Century?"*

As some of you know, I am studying towards a doctor of science degree. It so happens that the topic of my dissertation is also the topic of my newest book. Progress on that book is being delayed because "in between" I wrote yet another book that is also published "as we speak," *Kefir Rediscovered!* Yet another reason for a New Year's celebration. If you read *Kombucha Rediscovered!*, you will

---

* Richtungsweisend für die Therapie im 21. Jahrhundert? (Helfer Verlag, Großbuchhandlung Schwabe). The German-language book retails for $19.80 plus shipping/handling of $5.00. Readers who are interested in obtaining a copy of the German edition *Silicium – Heilung durch Ursubstanz* are invited to contact the author by faxing (604) 421-3610, emailing *Guileless@msn.com*, or by snail mail: 9566 Willowleaf Place, Burnaby, BC, V5A 4A5, Canada.

appreciate this book as the most *natural* successor. Anyway, I have been researching the field of electromagnetism for some time. And here's my dilemma! The deeper I look into electromagnetic phenomena, the more I get the uncanny feeling that electromagnetism and silica share a common denizen of the deepest significance. That common denominator may well turn out to be Professor Kervran's biological transmutation.

I think biological transmutation could well be the new medical miracle awaiting us in the new millennium. In this new edition therefore, I am reawakening that to me still somewhat nebulous power of transmuting. I will (almost) restrict myself to transmuting silica into other elements. See Chapter Nine: Biological Transmutation - Miracle of 2000 and Beyond. And now, happy reading!

Foreword

Let me give you the bad news first: the human body is a carbon/oxygen metabolic device that has come to the end of the line. As a species, we live on a planet that is over-populated, almost hopelessly polluted and starving for oxygen. It was less than a hundred years ago that the air on this planet was composed of nearly 40 percent oxygen. In the last decade of the 20th century, this figure is down to about 20 percent. The depletion of the ozone layer is really the result of low oxygen concentrations, not ozone destruction. After all, ozone is manufactured in nature from oxygen. No oxygen, no ozone layer.

We are rapidly running out of uncontaminated air, water and food. We still, as a species, eat far too many animals and animal products loaded with antibiotics, male and female hormones, cancer-causing chemicals and deadly, antibiotic-resistant microbes. Basic natural health education for the masses is still in its infancy. Some of the more obvious effects of all this are the cancer and AIDS pandemics, the exploding numbers of people suffering from chronic fatigue syndrome, total allergy disease and a long list of other immune system problems.

Conservative scientists estimate that one out of every three people in North America will get cancer during their lifetime. Most of this is not due directly to cigarette smoking but to chemical pollution and the low oxygen content of the air we breathe. It is 1997 and mainstream medicine continues to waste precious time treating HIV infections with an arsenal of dangerous and ineffective antiviral drugs. By the year 2000, over 120 million new cases of HIV infection are expected. The drugs are likely to have the same impact on HIV that the fiddle did for Nero as Rome burned to the ground.

Chronic fatigue syndrome now afflicts about 15 percent of the North American population. By the year 2000 this may triple. Every health care system in the world is finding it more and more difficult, if not impossible, to afford even basic band-aid treatments for the growing numbers of people suffering from degenerative diseases caused by diet, lifestyle and the environment. Health insurance is a myth simply because it has no direct health enhancement effects.

Now the good news: as *Homo sapiens* evolve to a different species fit enough to withstand the environmental pressures of the 21st century it will need the help of antioxidant nutrients. Without the antioxidant protection of high blood and tissue levels of vitamin A, beta carotene, vitamin C, E, selenium, zinc, silicon and others, the fragile carbon/oxygen human machinery cannot survive into the 21st century.

After reading this latest Klaus Kaufmann masterpiece, I am convinced that the most important of all the antioxidants is silica. Why? The answer is simple. Although our organic chemistry is based on the carbon atom, it could just as easily be based on silicon. As you will read in this well-researched book, this "final" step in human evolution may be a foregone conclusion. Carbon/oxygen replaced by silicon/oxygen? Yes, it may indeed come to pass.

It is an undisputed fact that healthy people have blood vessels and other tissues with greater levels of silicon than those suffering from degenerative diseases. Will a process of natural selection create a new type of human being operating as a silicon/oxygen organism? Science implies that it is within the realm of possibility.

Healthy people do not pick up infections with innocuous viruses like HIV, the chronic fatigue syndrome virus (whatever it turns out to be) and generally non-pathogenic fungi like candida albicans. Although no one can guarantee that all degenerative and immune system diseases can be prevented with a daily silica or silica gel supplement, Kaufmann will convince you that the survival odds are definitely in favor of those who do.

Aside from the use of silica for longevity and disease prevention, Kaufmann clearly details all of the many therapeutic uses of silica and silica gel. Some of the case histories he describes underline the versatility of this vital, yet low profile essential mineral. Brittle nails, hair loss, osteoporosis, degenerative disc disease, atherosclerosis, coronary artery disease, cancer, diabetes, aging, gastritis, ulcers, recurrent infections, skin disorders and a long list of other health problems can respond favorably to high doses of silica gel. It is quite possible that what you are about to read will save your life or the life of a loved one.

Zoltan P. Rona, M.D., M.Sc.
The *alive* Advisor and
author of *Return to the Joy of Health*

"I shall probably not live to witness the importance that the colloid chemistry of siliceous matter will play in the not too distant future. Colloid chemistry of matter containing silicon as its major component will become a serious competitor to organic chemistry as it is now defined, and therefore deserves far more attention than it now receives."

Rudolf Wegscheider, Ph.D.
Head of the First Chemical Institute
of the University of Vienna, Austria
October 1919

Introduction

The health secrets and therapeutic workings of an amazing mineral silica dispersed in a gel-like preparation are the topic of this book. Though silica was fashioned by nature millions of years ago, only in the past few years have we learned (and are learning still!) that its key element of silicon is vital and essential to building and maintaining living organisms. Extensive scientific research conducted in the USA, Germany and the former USSR has confirmed that silicon is a fundamental key to prevention of disease and to the maintenance of health. More amazingly still is the crucial role silica plays in gerontology and the prevention of premature aging.

In the fall of 1990 I was having great fun presenting signed hardcovers of my book on spring horsetail entitled *Silica – The Forgotten Nutrient* at the Convention Centre adjoining the Empress Hotel in sunny Victoria, BC. In between chatting with visitors to our booth, I found a few moments for surveying other exhibits. My eyes became glued to a new product exhibited right across from our booth. It was an odorless and odor-adsorbent foot powder. The exhibitor informed me that the foot powder traps bacterial molecules and that it thus eliminates unpleasant foot odor. In a confidential tone, he added, "This is nothing other than mineral silica in powdered form. Without any additives," he proudly emphasized, "it is totally non-poisonous and eco-friendly." His comments reminded me that I had not found the time for investigating silica gel, though, because of the great importance it has, I had promised myself to somehow fit it into my, at the time, very hectic schedule. As if on cue, the man from across the aisle sounded into my reveries, "You know, of course, that you could eat this powder and eradicate all kinds of ailments, not just eliminate foot odor." I had to smile. Animals like chickens or dogs could perhaps digest raw mineral silica, but humans? Even if he ate his mineral silica powder, it could not be assimilated very well by his metabolism. Ordinary powdered mineral silica is hardly edible and would be very difficult to absorb.

Nevertheless, the talk fuelled my determination. On returning from Victoria, I tackled the translation of a field study that had been done with a product derived from mineral silica. I had mentioned this study briefly in the first silica volume. I left it out because it did not fall within the scope of a work on horsetail. I had received numerous requests for the text of the field study.

Well, here it is finally. It makes up most of chapter seven. The individual patient's rehabilitations, because of their immediacy and the connection to real people, convinced me of silica gel's therapeutic powers more than anything else. The study chosen is best reflective of the general sweep of other case studies on silica gel. In fact, the recovery rates of all empirical evidence on silica gel is remarkably similar. I include an overview of the other studies done with silica gel at the beginning of Chapter Seven– The Healing Journey of 73 in '72.

This account of silica gel completes my investigation of silica. As this work does not use chemical formulas extensively, explanations of terminology will help to avoid ambiguity. Several terms relating to the element silicon are in common use. Silicon has a great affinity for and easily combines with oxygen. Not surprisingly, the most commonly found silicon compound is the oxide of silicon called silicon dioxide (SiO_2). It is best known as quartz that is made up of one silicon atom bound to two oxygen atoms in a three atom molecule. This compound is generally called silica.

Organic silica from horsetail and gelatinous mineral silica, i.e., "silica gel," the subject of this book, are dietary forms in which essential elementary silicon can be made available as a mineral supplement for human consumption. After processing of the raw material plant stock, organic vegetal silica consists mainly of SiO_2. The nutrient "silica gel" is also made up mainly of SiO_2, but stems from a pure mineral crystal source and has a chemical composition that uniquely assists the metabolizing of silica in the human alimentary canal.

Much of our present knowledge on silica comes from Germany where silica is called "Kieselsäure." This translates into "silicic acid" rather than "silica," the term commonly used in nutrition in North America. Scientific terminology clarified in 1955 by Ernst A. Hauser, Ph.D., Sc.D., Professor of Colloid Science at the Massachusetts Institute of Technology, denotes "colloidal silicic acid" (H_4SiO_4) as a fluid mixture containing hydrated silica, i.e., silicon dioxide that is associated with hydrogen and/or water molecules. The term "silica gel," as used in this work, does not refer to the hardened, dried and roasted industrial dehydrated, desiccated silica gel that chemical industry uses as a drying agent for gases and organic solvents.

To be precise, within the context of this work, the term "silica gel" denotes a dietary colloidal preparation of silica in an active, highly dispersed form in purified water. The fascinating steps from quartz crystal to silica gel are detailed in chapter two – Heaven is a Colloidal. The colloidal condition makes clear why dietary silica gel can boost the immune system to such a degree that it even offers hope for sufferers from today's new immune deficiency diseases.

Super-versatile silica gel offers not only therapy from within and without simultaneously, it also plays an ever greater role in daily nutrition because of the increasingly precarious equilibrium our bodies must maintain to assure continued health and disease prevention against a backdrop of a constantly deteriorating environment. So it is pertinent, if surprising, that silica is also essential for the production and renewal of the life-giving oxygen we all breathe every second of our lives. Even better, silica was instrumental in creating the very first step that made the development of life on our planet possible.

While this work contains all health applications of silica gel known to me, through the use of their own inventive imagination, readers will no doubt discover new effective uses for silica gel. And now, I invite my readers to follow me on a very personal and scintillating journey. The search for the source of silica gel takes us all the way back to my childhood paradise.

Chapter One

"Every secret knowledge gleaned from Nature, without scientific illumination and empirical validation, in the end degenerates into superstition, prejudice, and mental darkness."
Christoph Wilhelm Hufeland*

Origins of a Malleable Mineral of Strength and Vitality

The Secret of the White Sand

I spent a great part of my childhood and youth exploring the pure white sands of the Lüneburger Heide. I often came here looking for small animals I could add to my terrarium. The Heide (Lunenburg Heath in English) surrounds my native city of Hannover in Germany. The seemingly motionless heath is the eerie, lonely and often foggy flatland that makes up much of the Province of Lower Saxony. The region is so flat and so close to sea level that in the '50s great stretches of it were flooded when a gigantic tornado broke the dykes of the North Sea and swept the waters of the Atlantic Ocean onto the heath. I wrote a poem about that cataclysm.

When I was a child, I believed the white sand fields near my home to be the offshoots and runners of the beautiful white sand dunes gracing the East Frisian Islands off the German North Atlantic coast. From their adjoining tidelands, mud flats expand into the lonely hinterland of the heath. You would not know to look at it (I certainly did not then!), but

* Translated from the German by Klaus Kaufmann.

5

the white sand of the heath is the natural raw material for the medicinal silica gel that, as we will discover, can positively affect diverse ailments from light skin conditions to the most dreadful silent killer disease – atherosclerosis.[*]

Essential Body Functions of Silica Gel

It is perhaps fitting that the most abundant elements fulfill some of the most vital tasks within the human body. These elements are silicon and oxygen. Together they make up silica. Understanding the ins and outs of oxygen inside the human body is as easy as breathing in and breathing out. Oxygen is present in the living body in large quantities. Contrariwise, the second most abundant element on earth after oxygen, silicon, is present in the body only as a trace element, amounting to no more than perhaps 15 micrograms per 100 ml of body fluid. Why would this be so?

One reason might be that in unassisted form silica, the compound of silicon, is rather insoluble. This explains why we do not take in much of it despite its universal abundance. Yet research conducted by Professor Edith Carlisle at UCLA and others shows silicon to be involved in very important and metabolic as well as structural processes in higher animals and human beings. As will be shown, her 1972 studies show silicon to be an essential trace element, just as essential as, for instance, vitamin C.

In order to qualify for the appellation of "essential," an element must show a reproducible effect on a vital process in the living body that cannot occur without the element. The element silicon facilitates essential processes that go on only in the presence of silicon. These processes stop if silicon is withdrawn. The processes are restored when silicon is added again. Such reproducible studies performed "in vitro" and/or "in vivo" verify that silicon is an essential element.

[*] In Europe more commonly named "arteriosclerosis."

Dr. Carlisle* confirmed silicon as an essential element. During a conversation I had with her, she pointed out that it took science so long to identify silicon as an essential trace element because it occurs in such very low levels in the blood and tissue. She pointed out that older silicon research was complicated by the fact that silicon "in vitro" studies innocently used glass vials. Glass, of course, consisting of mainly silica, tends to distort findings on silicon. This was overcome by switching to silicon-free lab equipment. But why is silicon essential?

A quick countdown of silicon's important uses in the human body reveals that it:
- stimulates cell metabolism and cell formation.
- inhibits the aging process in tissues. Younger people's tissues always show a higher silica content.
  Unsupported, the silica content decreases with age. This has been corroborated with tests done on the tissues of the human aorta.
- is important for both the structure and the functioning of connective tissue. Silica deficiency leads to the weakening of connective tissue.
- increases elasticity and firmness of blood vessels. This helps to avoid arteriosclerotic conditions. As the arteries' elastic connective tissue is rejuvenated (elasticized with silica), the arteriosclerotic deswelling vanishes.
- is anti-inflammatory, disinfecting, absorbing and odor-binding.
- stimulates the immune system to help the body fight off disease-causing intruders.

Nature's Most Perfect Energizer
Our immune system is the most crucial protective function

* Dr. Carlisle's "in vitro" and "in vivo" research that is mentioned throughout this text was based on a scientifically purified silicon free of any other elementary traces. It was specifically prepared for research purposes in the form of pure sodium metasilicate. Dr. Carlisle makes it clear that sodium metasilicate is not intended and not recommended as a supplement to human nutrition.

our body owns. Without it, we die. Silica gel activates the immune function. It helps to create the matrix that enables the body to fight off infections and environmental toxins. Silica gel mobilizes the body's defenses against foreign intruders and disease-causing micro-organisms.

The immunity system boosting effect has been confirmed. If for no other reason, we would need a silica supplement for body armor. But unlike a purely defensive force, silica gel also builds up the body. This is good news for those interested in body building. The sports-medicinal anabolic "formula" of silica gel is legal and, unlike steroids, improves your health.

One would think that the therapeutic benefits of silica should have become common knowledge over the years. Yet, it is true even now that only herbal practitioners, naturopaths and homeopaths seriously consider silica as a bio-healer. Official medicine hardly even mentions silica in pharmacological textbooks. If the media ever broadcast the therapeutic effects of silica, it could quickly become the preventive therapy of choice.

Thirty years ago, silica researcher Hugo Schulz strongly complained about orthodox medicine's ignorance of silica in his native Germany. His urging was not in vain. The German authorities wrote silica into the new edition of the pharmacological textbook of Germany – a tremendous victory of right over might. It started the search for an effective supplementary silica formula.

All the body's connective tissues need silica. This was verified by the research done by Dr. Carlisle of the School of Public Health, University of California. Dr. Carlisle found that low concentrations of silicon in most organs, with the exception of the lungs, do not vary appreciably during life. It follows that the organs can fulfill their myriad functions only when daily doses of 20 to 30 mg of silica (containing silicon) are constantly provided (this is equivalent to 0.308 to 0.463 grains). Because of this constant consumption, the effective or working silica content of living organisms is linked irreversibly to diet.

Shouldn't a priceless energizer like silica be rare? Not at all. Earth's outer crust consists mainly of silica. Yet, silica deficiencies and consequent ailments are common, as common as oxygen starvation occurring, for instance, in cancerous cells with oxygen in abundance in surrounding tissue. This enigma of universal oversupply and cellular underutilization makes it so important to replenish essential body silica to prevent or treat deficiencies. Before we can take a closer look at specific silica gel applications, let us have a look at its underpinning element – silicon.

Silicon's Similarity and Rivalry with Carbon
Silicon, having a great affinity for oxygen, oxidizes rapidly to form silica. For this reason silicon is never found as the free element. Silica, the dioxide of silicon, is therefore the main topic of this work. However, silicon has wide applications in technology. New, ever more exciting silicon research is under way. Much of it is directed at health improvement via technology.

One such new application melds biology and electronics in detection devices known as biosensors. Silicon-supported biosensors are intended to replace animal testing, bestowing "humanitarian" qualities on silicon. Another application involves electrorheological fluids that transform rapidly from a lubricant to a solid and back again. In this, dielectric particles are suspended in silicon.

There's seemingly no limit to silicon's technological uses. Silicon's great range of uses makes it similar to the range of carbon. As you may know, organic chemistry got its label of "organic" from carbon. (This use of "organic" does not refer to the organic fertilizer used in natural farming, of course.) Silicon is in the same group as carbon in the periodic system of elements. Does this explain silicon's bioavailability? Perhaps.

The Periodic Table classifies elements according to their atomic number. The table is divided into horizontal and vertical rows, according to atomic structure. Elements that are placed close to each other in the Periodic Table closely resemble each other in nature. Silicon, atomic number 14, is placed directly below carbon in the Periodic Table. This placement in the fourth group confirms that of all the elements, silicon – the element of mineral chemistry – is the most similar to carbon, the element of organic chemistry.

Silicon is usually tetravalent like carbon in its organic compounds. This valency* is significant. Both of these elements are vital to sustaining life. Carbon is the most important ingredient in vitamin C and, of course, the carbohydrates in food. I will relate an interesting story concerning vitamin C and its discoverer and the silicon connection to vitamin C. You will find that silicon and carbon's vitamin C are mutually beneficial. This is perhaps not too surprising. The element silicon has now become a serious competitor of organic chemistry, giving rise to a new branch of science called "silicic chemistry."

Two Elements Rule the Earth
Among the many elements making up the earth's crust, silicon holds an outstanding position. Although, as pointed out in the introduction, in its pure atomic or elementary form, silicon cannot exist on earth, it abounds in bonded forms. We

---

* Valency (also valence) is the property possessed by an element or radical of combining with or replacing other elements or radicals in definite and constant proportion.

can say that, while on earth, silicon always needs a partner. It bonds and by that bonding process it changes its name.

But silicon very seldom bonds in its simplest salt-like form. Most often, it forms multi-nuclear structures known as oxo-complexes. It also forms the natural and technologically important silicates. The more complex silicates take on a more diamond-like character with quartz as its final link. Silicon usually occurs in oxygenated rocks or in quartz, sand and clay.

Silicon's bonding with oxygen is very fitting. Together these two elements rule the earth. Silicon takes part in 40 percent, almost half, of the formation of the earth's crust. This makes silicon the second most abundant element on our planet after oxygen. Oxygen, the primary element of life, makes up the other half weight of our earth. When the two most abundant elements on earth "marry," we can expect some awesome offsprings.

Hard as Rock is Wedlock
In its wedded state, silicon dioxide, now called silica, enters the mineral family of the silicates. The silicates are minerals composed of the elements of silicon and oxygen. They can bond with each other alone or they can combine with other elements, such as carbon. By now it may not surprise you to learn that the silicon element is so all-encompassing that almost all minerals are silicates. In fact, geology has found and classified more than 1,000 silicates to date. That is a massive preponderance for silica on earth, about 87 percent of earth's crust and about 26 percent of the outer portion of the earth.

More precisely, I should have said "in" the earth. Our planet's crust varies from 10 to 70 kilometers in thickness. The crusty shell is composed almost entirely of silicates. Beyond that, the surfaces of the moon and of Mars, and probably even the deeper mantle zone within the earth, are made of silicates. Little surprise then, that the most widely used construction materials – glass, ceramic, brick, concrete and much building stone – consist entirely or mainly of silicates.

What a Gem!

In the elementary silicon family, where there's abundance, there's also much beauty and great purity. Indeed, silicon's offsprings are awesome to behold even if they take a very long time to grow. An overwhelming majority of silica exists as quartz in crystalline or grown form. During their formation these crystals have been purified by nature. Silica gel originates from such wondrous quartz structures that are built up from silicon dioxide. Even more highly prized gems, such as emeralds, aquamarine and tourmaline, and also the more massive semiprecious stones like amethyst, rose quartz, agate, jasper, and chalcedony, are all made of silica.

What good would beauty alone be if it were not also useful? Silica is tremendously so for building and agriculture. Silica is the major constituent of light-colored igneous rocks such as granite, branddiorite, and quartz monzonite and their volcanic equivalents. If you are an aspiring geologist, you might be interested to know that of the silicates, cristobalite and trydymite are the most uncommon. Coesite, stishovite, vitreous silica, and melanophlogite are rare. Several other silica polymorphs have been synthesized in the lab. As quartz is resistant to mechanical and chemical weathering, it constitutes the bulk of shale and sandstone, the most common sedimentary rock types.

Silica in Hot Waters

Where crystals cannot go, dispersions can. Silica dispersion in silica-containing mineral waters varies between 70 mg/litre to 400 mg per liter. Given the abundance of silica stones and sand, it is not too amazing that most mineral waters contain silica. The Europeans found this out ages ago. Therapy with mineral waters is very popular in their exclusive spas and health retreats. A large part of the medicinal effect of mineral waters must be credited to the silica content of the waters.

Geyserite, or siliceous sinter, is a hydrous silica that is rapidly precipitated from cooling waters flowing away from geothermal springs and geysers. For example, the Wilhelms Spring in Kronthal near Frankfurt on Main, in Germany, contains 100 mg per liter, and the Marienbad Forest Spring 400 mg of silicic acid per liter. The famous Dunaris spring water in the German Eiffel show a content of 80 mg per litre. Other famous silica spas in Germany are: Teinacher Hirschquelle with 70 mg per liter, Glashäger Heilwasser with 70 mg per liter and Baden-Badener with 155 mg per liter. Other famous examples of silica-rich hot springs are found all around the globe: in Iceland, New Zealand and Yellowstone Park in the US.

Silica abundance in hot springs is due to silica minerals that can be transported in steam or in warm waters. At higher temperatures and pressures, fluids carry greater amounts of silica. Conversely, silica precipitates when cooling or pressure-release occurs. Things can work in reverse. It is often the hot waters that deposit quartz veins and the quartz gangue common in ore deposits.

Alzheimer's and the Ions of Silicon and Aluminum
In the natural silicates, multi-nuclear negatively charged complexes are held together by positive ions, called cations. One, feldspar, used in homeopathy, is a crystallized silicate. It is a silica salt that forms through the building of aluminum atoms in the neutral body network of silica. Aluminum ions, because they are similar in size to silicon ions, readily substitute for silicon ions in aluminosilicates.

Dr. Carlisle is currently doing research on the aluminum and silicon[*] interactions that promises to lead to exciting new discoveries such as a possible connection between aluminum and Alzheimer's that has not yet been established. Funded by California's Alzheimer's Foundation, Carlisle ran a study using old female rats equivalent in age to humans around 70. When put on a low silicon diet, these rats tended to accumulate aluminum in the brain. When put on a high silicon diet, they did not accumulate aluminum in the brain!

Research is ongoing. No conclusions have been arrived at, but it promises to be very interesting. Meanwhile, the interim results show that the element sought regarding a possible connection to Alzheimer's concerns aluminum and not silicon.[†] As we can gather, on investigating a broad range remedy like silica, a good guide map is fundamental to finding your way. Otherwise chances are that you will miss the right turn.

Biological Transmutation Revisited
Researcher E. Lemberg, in studying the behavior of fertilizers in soil in 1876, found that ion exchange was reversible and stoichiometric. This mouthful of a word applies to elements that can be chemically combined by weight and volume. At the time, the reversibility and combining power was earth-shattering news. It meant, for example, that one mole of sodium could replace one mole of potassium.

Around 1900, scientists discovered that complex hydrous sodium and potassium aluminum silicates (zeolites), could

---

[*] Headed "Aluminum and silicon," on page 132 and 133 of the book *Encyclopedia of Natural Medicine,* (1991), Prime Publishing, CA, USA, authors Michael Murray, ND, and Joseph Pizzorno, ND, infer silicon as possibly co-causative in Alzheimer's. This has not been proven, which Pizzorno readily admitted. The text advocates reducing exposure to silicon. This is doubly misleading because: 1. Silicon is ubiquitous; avoiding exposure is nearly impossible, and 2. Silicon is an essential trace element in the human organism.

[†] The *Encyclopedia of Natural Medicine* suggests a connection to Alzheimer's for aluminum *and* silicon! According to Dr. Carlisle, this is absurd and based on incorrect interpretations of existing references.

exchange their sodium or potassium ions for calcium and similar ions if leached by a solution of those ions. Is there a possible connection here between the biological transmutation of silicon atoms into calcium atoms and the observed and well-known ion exchanges?

Though it was perhaps not realized at the time, these discoveries led to the theory of biological transmutation. The concept of biological transmutation, an apparently blatant contradiction to the laws of physics and chemistry, is the brainchild of Kervran. I have discussed its medical repercussions in great depth in the companion volume to this book, which I strongly recommend to interested readers.[3]

In High Form

Even in ancient times, "high forms" of silica crystals played a special role in the maintenance and restoration of people's health. When temperatures are increased, the atomic linkages in quartz undergo a tilting without causing any structural disruption. This process causes forms with higher symmetry. Such constructs are called "high forms." In ancient times such quartz crystals held a special charm and attraction mainly for ornamental reasons. However, a tribal shaman, perhaps instinctively sensing the healthful value of silica, used quartz for magical-medical incantations.

In the American Indians' spiritual and health rituals, the Medicine Wheel played an important part. The wheel held a quartz crystal—the hidden "power object." The Indians said that, "in the body of the Earth Mother, crystals are akin to the brain cells. Gemstones are the organs, rocks the muscles, sand the skin, and trees or foliage the hair." Not surprisingly, crystals became a symbol of the spirit and of the intellect in association with the spirit.

Today quartz crystals are the hidden power objects in modern watches, keeping time with their internal vibrations. No matter, quartz, even without ethical and magical attributes, is the most useful of the silica minerals. It has hundreds of other commercial uses. Crushed quartz stone and sand are part of the ingredients for concrete and mortar, in refractories, foundry molds, ceramics, glass, silicon carbide, silicon metal, fluxes for melting, abrasives, and in sandblasting.

As though that is not enough, high-purity quartz has application in the making of vitreous silica, which has very low thermal expansion, high elasticity, and transparency to light qualities. This makes vitreous silica desirable for lenses, optical fibers, components of precision instruments, and premium grades of chemical glassware. All this constitutes ample proof that silica quartz contains an abundance of energy for applications. Yet there is more still.

Icicles' Crystalline Delight
Things often are not what they appear to be. The icicles of wintry days are a perfect example. In the water molecule's crystallization process, hydrogen (instead of silicon) bonds with oxygen. Imagine, if aliens saw ice for the first time, would they know they beheld water in a frozen state or would they think they had discovered a new type of transparent hard rock or precious stone? Would they know that the air in which they were immersed was saturated with the essence of that ice in its gaseous form? As they inclined over a spring to taste the refreshing liquid bubbling forth, would they realize that its silky softness was that same element that they found as a crystalline rock?

The world is full of surprises like that. As water is to ice, so silica gel is to quartz. The quartz crystal has a precisely balanced, uniform internal atomic structure. Silica crystals hold and transmit energy. Their widespread use for maintaining exact timing is an aspect of this ability. If silica's artful and timely performance in technology does so impress, perhaps its power and purpose in biochemistry is just as impressive? But before returning to silica gel's role within living tissue, we need to find out about the nature of gels.

Chapter Two

"The flint particles remain suspended in the
liquid and at the same time invisible, due to
their fineness and transparency."

Torbern Bergman, Ph.D.
Siliceous Researcher, 1779

Heaven is a Colloidal

A Scattering of Blue

Asking why the sky is blue was my standard question to vex
adults when I was six years old. I was driving my parents to
distraction by forever asking questions for which they did
not have answers. My valiant father told me that dust in the
upper atmosphere reflects light from the sun, and that
mainly the color blue is reflected, which is why the sky
looks blue. His answer satisfied me only for a time. I don't
like to say so, but my father was not quite right. We will
detour a little to the chemical and physical behavior of
small particles to find the right answer and to discover more
about silica gel.

A scattering of small particles of matter dispersed in a
liquid, gas, or solid is called a "colloid." This term comes
from a Greek word for "glue." But it is not glue that holds
them together. Milk, smoke, and fog are also common
examples of colloids. So is ink.

As a boy I used to have fun watching colloidal dispersion of
ink drops. I would pour tap water into my mother's tall
crystal vase. Then I waited until the water in the vase was

motionless. Then I squeezed a droplet of ink from my fountain pen and let it fall into the water. For a while the ink would sink rapidly. Then it would start to disperse into an upside down smoke stack and slowly form the most interesting shapes. Eventually it dispersed evenly throughout the water. The fun was over.

The size of a particle determines whether or not it qualifies as a colloid. Too large and it doesn't, too small and it doesn't. To measure the size of a particle in a colloid, a unit of distance called the angstrom is used. An angstrom unit, named after a Swedish physicist, is a unit of length equal to 10^{-8} cm, i.e., one angstrom unit (abbreviated Å). One Å is equal to the diameter of a hydrogen atom. The colloidal range of matter consists of particles measuring from 10 to 10,000Å. That confirms that colloids are very small particles that are held in solution.

A colloid is not a true solution however, such as a solution of sugar or salt. In a true solution, the particles are even smaller. A particle of a true solution is a small molecule composed of just a few atoms. It can also be an ion, an electrically charged particle. Colloidal particles are usually united in a small crystalline aggregate or joined to form a long, stringy molecule. Colloidal particles, though fine enough to pass through ordinary filter paper, are large enough to be separated from the solvent by the processes of ultrafiltration and ultracentrifugation. Particles of a true solution, however, being about the same size as the molecules of the solvent, cannot be separated by any type of filtration or centrifugation, not even ultrafiltration and ultracentrifugation.

On the upper side of matter particles, the difference between a colloid such as ink, and a coarse dispersion, such as muddy water, is that colloidal particles are so much smaller. The influence of gravity tending to separate them out is inconsequential compared with the scattering forces that keep the colloidal particles dispersed. Consequently, particles of a colloid have little or no tendency to settle out. In contrast, the relatively large particles of coarse dispersions separate spontaneously in a short time by gravitational migration to the bottom or top of the medium, depending on the medium and the specific gravity of the particles.

The properties of colloids are so unlike those of either true solutions or coarse dispersions and play such a prominent role in natural processes of both living and nonliving matter that an independent branch of knowledge, colloid science, has resulted from the study of the colloidal state.

Colloids of solid particles are called "sols," solid sols, or aerosols, depending on whether the dispersion happens in a liquid, solid, or gas. The particles may also be liquid or gas, that is, droplets or bubbles of colloidal dimensions. This is best illustrated by a table that compares colloids of different dispersed particle phases and different mediums.

Name of Colloid	Dispersed Particle Phase	Medium	Examples
Sol	solid	liquid	ink, glue
Solid sol	solid	solid	steel, emerald
Aerosol	solid	gas	smoke, dust
Emulsion	liquid	liquid	milk, mayonnaise
Solid emulsion	liquid	solid	pearl, opal
Aerosol (liquid)	liquid	gas	fog, mist
Foam	gas	liquid	meringue, froth
	gas	gas	pumice, lava
			(no colloid possible)
Condensed colloid	solid	none	rubber, cotton

If both the dispersed particles and the medium is a gas, a colloid is not possible. Of all types of colloids, sols are by far the most important. They are divided into two large sub-groups, depending on whether they are (1) molecular sols, single giant molecules dispersed in a liquid, or (2) micellar sols, which are aggregates of small molecules, ions, or atoms dispersed in a liquid. Most organic sols – sols of proteins, cellulose, starch, rubber and synthetic polymers – are molecular sols.

Single molecule (molecular) sols can usually be prepared merely by adding the solid material to the appropriate liquid; for example, a sol of milk proteins is prepared by mixing powdered skim milk with water. The smaller the particles, the more transparent the sol is. A sol becomes usually transparent if the particles are more or less round and less than 300Å in diameter. If the particles are between 300Å and 5,000Å, the sol is opalescent, scattering a small portion of available light in all directions.

Thus we have rearrived at the sky of blue above, because scattering, once known as the Tyndall effect, is not caused by reflection from the surfaces of the particles like my father thought. Reflection from colloidal particles is not possible because they are smaller than the wavelength of visible light, which is from 3,500Å to 7,000Å. Since scattering of light is inversely proportional to the wavelength, blue light (short wavelength) is scattered more than red light (long wavelength). Consequently, when white light is scattered, the scattered light takes on a bluish tinge.

Many sols, like silica sols, look bluish white or blue when illuminated with white light and viewed from a direction perpendicular to the direction of incident light. One of the most striking scattering of light effects involving silica is iridescence, the effect observed with opals. In fact, opals are the fossilized remains of an earlier colloidal crystal suspension!

Ordinary small molecules as well as colloidal particles scatter light, but the intensity of scattering by tiny molecules is so weak that it is not noticeable except in the deep layers of water and air that constitute clear lakes and skies. The scattered light is predominantly blue, and even in these relatively pure media much of the scattering is caused by such colloidal particles as dust and micro-organisms.

The Sol of Silica
The particles of different sols have shapes that vary from spheres to slender threads. Particles of gold and many other micellar sols are more or less globular or polyhedral. Because such particles can pass by one another with ease, the viscosity of these sols is only slightly greater than the viscosity of the liquid in which they are dispersed.

On the other hand, sols containing thread-like particles become tangled whenever the liquid is disturbed. A sol of ordinary rubber cement is highly viscous even if it contains only one percent rubber, since a rubber molecule is about 30,000Å long and only a few angstroms thick. Egg white, a sol of albumin in water, is of intermediate viscosity because the albumin molecule, although very long, is coiled into a ball of globular protein. A silica sol closely resembles the albumin character of egg white and another sol, human blood.

The Solvation Army
Colloidal particles show varying degrees of affinity for the liquid in which they are dispersed. If the affinity is high, molecules of the liquid are tightly affixed to the surface and are even incorporated inside the particle. The particle can thus be considered as swollen and composed of a mixture of solid and liquid. A sol containing such particles is a lyophilic (solvent-loving) sol. Examples are water glass (polysilicic acid dispersed in water), glue, and rubber in benzene.

Crystalline particles, such as those in sulphur sols (milk of sulphur) and gold sols (drinkable gold) are not highly solvated, that is, are not dissolved to any great extent, and are said to be lyophobic (solvent-hating). The degree of solvation of a particle depends to some extent on its shape; threadlike particles tend to be lyophilic because of their relatively large surface area.

A Perpetual State of Suspension

Colloidal particles are held in a perpetual state of suspension by the continuous bombardment they receive from the surrounding molecules of liquid. This bombardment is a consequence of the ordinary thermal motion of molecules. The average velocity of a single water molecule at room temperature is about 1,400 miles per hour. When a coarse particle is struck on all sides by millions of these fast-moving molecules each second, no net momentum is imparted to the particle.

If the particle is very small, however, fluctuations in the impacts on opposite sides are significant, with the result that the particle is jostled first in one direction, then in another. A colloidal particle placed in a liquid or gas is subject to Brownian movement, a ceaseless, random motion. Most sols would have but a momentary existence, however, if coalescence of the particles were not prevented. The small particles on colliding would otherwise stick together, and would soon grow to such size that the rate of sedimentation would become large as compared with the rate of Brownian movement. Accretion of the colloidal particle of stable sols is prevented by adsorbed substances, especially by adsorbed ions.

The affinity of a solid for an ion depends on the nature of the solid and on the size, charge, and chemical properties of the ion. When placed in a solution containing different types of ions, a solid particle selectively adsorbs some of the ions and acquires a charge of the sign of the ion for which it has the greatest affinity.

As a result of selective adsorption the particles all carry a charge of the same sign and consequently repel one another. The force of repulsion between two particles is negligible if they are more than a few angstroms apart; but when the distance becomes less and collision is imminent, the force of repulsion increases to such an extent that actual contact between the particles is prevented. The stability of many sols depends on the kind and amount of ions present.

The ions adsorbed on the surface or part of the surface of every colloidal particle attract ions of the opposite charge to the vicinity of the particle. These counter ions form a cloud around the particle called the diffuse outer layer. By screening the particle, the diffuse outer layer reduces its effective charge. This phenomenon is so pronounced when the concentration of ions is high that the charges on the particles are no longer effective in preventing collisions. Low concentrations of electrolytes stabilize a sol; high concentrations destroy it.

A Gel with a Sol
When egg white (albumen) is heated, the weak bonds that hold the coils together break, the molecule unfolds, and the sol becomes viscous. When fully extended, the albumin molecules are so tangled and interlocked that the egg white is a semi-solid: a gel. The unfolding of protein molecules under the influence of heat is a general phenomenon; it is assumed to be the chief event of denaturation and a principal cause of death to organisms by heat.

A gel is a sol in which the particles are branched and interlocked threads. A jelly is defined as a gel that contains an especially large proportion of liquid. When the liquid of a gel is removed by evaporation, surface tension forces pull the fibers together, causing the network structure to collapse. The result, a zerogel, is typified by a sheet of dry gelatine. Replacing the liquid with air without collapsing the gel produces an aerogel, which is soft, nearly transparent, and extremely light. Now that we have an understanding of colloids and sols and gels, we can return the discussion to the making of silica gel.

The Polymerization of Silica or Bonds of Fundamental Importance to Life

In order to become a colloidal silica gel, silica, in the form of orthosilicic acid (H_4SiO_4), must first polymerize. Silicic acid, under elimination of water, polymerizes into three-dimensional polysilicas formed from several molecules. Polymerization is the chemical term for a reaction that results in successively larger molecules. These eventually result in long chains, thus:

$$
\begin{array}{ccccccc}
OH & & OH & & & OH & OH \\
| & & | & & & | & | \\
HO\text{-}Si\text{-}OH & + & HO\text{-}Si\text{-}OH & - & H_2O + & HO\text{-}Si\text{-}O\text{-}Si\text{-}OH \\
| & & | & \longrightarrow & & | & | \\
OH & & OH & & & OH & OH
\end{array}
$$

If you look closely, you can soon see how in such a chain, each oxygen ion serves as a partner for two silicon ions, ie,

$$
\begin{array}{cc}
O & O \\
| & | \\
O\text{-}Si\text{-}O\text{-}Si\text{-}O \\
| & | \\
O & O
\end{array}
$$

Such four-sided chain links are called tetrahedra. This term comes from a Greek word for a four-sided figure. In other words, SiO_2 is a network of SiO_4 tetrahedra. As can be seen, in this network each silicon atom is tetrahedrally surrounded by four oxygen atoms, each of which simultaneously belongs to two adjoining tetrahedra. The silicon atoms are thus all bound with one another through bridges made of oxygen. This linking of oxygen and silicon is a first step towards silica gel. The next step involves the chemical compound H_2O, much better known as water.

Water and the Sol-Gel Reversibility
In nature, silica occurs only as a water-free compound and in salt forms known as silicates. Water-binding silica, also called hydrous silica, arises from the freeing of silica from the water soluble alkaline silicates. Solid silica particles in a finely subdivided form enter into such an intimate mixture with water that the silica seems to dissolve in the water.

The watery solution is, however, not a real fusing like the solution of common table salt (sodium chloride) in water. When you mix table salt and water, you obtain a solution in which the sodium chloride disappears altogether as a solid compound. Solid silica particles, on the other hand, enter a mixture with water in a midway condition between solid and fluid. This intermediary dispersion of silica in water is a colloidal system in which the molecules are suspended rather than dissolved.

The relative quantities of the two portions of a colloidal system can determine whether the system has a sol (liquid) or a gel (solid) consistency. For example, if a small amount of protein, such as gelatin, is placed in water, a sol results; but if a large amount of gelatin is placed in water, then a gel results. This holds true also vis-a-vis other fluids and solids.

Therefore, in the human bloodstream silica is in a hydrosol (liquid hydrate of silicic acid) condition. In human nails, skin or hair, it takes on a hydrogel (gelatinous hydrate of silicic acid) condition. These twin colloidal powers of silica gel make it extremely adaptable. It makes colloidal silica gel valuable for external applications as well as for internal uses. So, silica gel adapts to the environment it finds itself in.

One of the biochemical advantages of colloidal silica is that it has such a huge surface for reacting. Silica gel's surface capacity is astounding. Just one gram boasts a surface of some 300 square meters! Put geometrically, it means that one cubic inch of gel possesses a surface area of 50,000 square feet. Or, if you could line up the particles in a row, the resultant distance would correspond with seventeen times the distance from the earth to the moon. Such a colossal surface activity of silica is of fundamental significance for the activation of living tissue. It gives colloidal silica gel great absorptive power.

Colloidal silica's surface tension is so unusually great, it increases exceptionally. Not only boundary surfaces between liquid and air exist, but also between silica and water. Thus, silica gel contains inner energies, and is, because of its very large surface activity, a fundamental condition for biological processes. We can now understand why the white silica sands of the Lunenburg Heath are of value in human health and nutrition.

Chapter Three

"In science the credit goes to the man who convinces the world, not to the man to whom the idea first occurs."

Sir William Osler, M.D.

Astounding Account of a Body Builder

The Milling of the White Sand

The white sand, of course, consists of pure quartz crystals that were ground to dust by receding mountains of ice that covered this part of the world eons ago during the so-called Ice Ages. Under the white quartz sand and in elevated areas, quartz crystals are today quarried from the surrounding rock. Recognized for their nutrient and curative value, these quarried crystal extracts are transported to a nearby factory where they are successively cleansed, milled and pulverised into a very fine powder. Next, the finely powdered and washed silica particles are suspended in a liquid by adding a brine solution. It is during the succeeding stage that the silica is precipitated out of this solution with the assistance of mineral acids.

After this stage the resultant silicic acid is sometimes still lumpy and is further homogenized until the resultant silicic acid-anhydride* has a uniform structure. For the processing, only purified, aseptic water is used. During a special

---

* An anhydride is a substance derived from a compound by the removal of water.

29

washing, hydrochloric acid is removed in a careful step-by-step process. Sodium chloride that was generated is separated from the sought-after silicic acid.

The ongoing process precipitates the silicic acid from the solution. Fresh water is added again and the washing process is repeated. This is done up to 12 times. The milling to microscopic particles eventually yields a continuous liquid substance in which the particles aggregate but do not settle or settle extremely slowly.

The resultant system is now no longer either a solution or a suspension – it is a colloid with a gel-like molecular scaffolding that is very similar in structure and appearance to the albuminoid arrangement of raw egg white. This albuminoid character of silica gel becomes quickly noticeable on use.

Not only does the gel look like egg white, it feels like it, too. When applying silica gel to the skin, the gel causes a tautening of the skin on drying just like egg white would. This is because in colloidal silica the silicon dioxide molecules (each molecule made up of one silicon atom and two oxygen atoms) are enveloped by water molecules (H_2O). This composition prevents molecular clustering. It eases passage through the intestines and enables the placement of active silicic acid into the body's connective tissues. Simultaneously, the gel formation allows the external and internal therapeutic application of silica.

What has happened is that the silica underwent a kind of "chelating" that helps assimilation on ingestion of silica gel. The individual silicon atoms are bound in finest colloidal dispersion (see chapter two for a full explanation of "colloidal"). This colloidal dispersion eases assimilation because of the great surface area that exists for the biochemical interaction between the human metabolism and the individual silica particles.

I pointed out in my first silica book that most mineral silica is not suitable for human consumption. Coarse fragments of raw silica (sand) are far too abrasive for the delicate human palate. Impurities present in such silica could be hazardous to human health.* The important processes described that yield colloidal silica gel must be undertaken first for even the purest of mineral silicas to achieve ease of absorption.

The Silica Gel Pioneer

The great role silica plays in therapy was forecast as early as 1878 by the famous French chemist and bacteriologist Louis Pasteur. The prophetic Pasteur pronouncement regarding silica was known to Dr. Becker, a German chemist who first formulated therapeutic silica gel. Dr. Becker was a former employee of the pharmaceutical giant I. G. Farben (now Hoechst) in Germany. He became interested in silica research at the end of World War II and studied all the available silica literature.

Dr. Becker became fascinated with the healing properties of silica and decided to develop a therapeutic from silica. He found that the watery form of the oxygen compound of silicic acid was best suited for his purposes. He formulated a product that became known as "Original Silicea Balsam." (It still is called so in Germany and in Canada. In the USA it has become known by the trade name of "Body Essential Silica Gel.") Dr. Becker's product is silicic acid that is precipitated into finest dispersion until it falls into a gel form. Dr. Becker, though schooled in pharmaceuticals and pre-

---

* While writing the manuscript to this book, my wife and I got a puppy. We named him Bing. I found it most curious that whenever we took Bing to the beaches he ate sand. When on meadows, he searched out and ate horsetail plants. It took some time before I figured him out. He needed extra silica for his thick coat and growing frame! To confirm this, I checked his dog food. Sure enough, the list of ingredients did not include silica.

scription medicines, developed his silica remedy primarily as a self-help therapeutic in natural health care.

Dr. Becker found that the individual molecules in his silica balsam would cluster into groups and that this yielded a gel of adsorbent and anti-inflammatory properties that could be used in healing cuts and bruises. This suited his goal of a therapeutic intended for internal and external uses. The product became quickly popular in Germany even before silicon had been recognized as an essential trace mineral.* Dr. Becker could not possibly know at the time that with the discovery – beginning in 1972 – of silicon as an essential trace element, the possible health applications of his balsam would spiral tremendously.

He might have known, however, of the application of siliceous bentonite gels for the healing of cuts and other skin injuries. Crude silica-rich bentonite gels were used by native Indians of the United States for generations. Dr. Becker also knew that an entirely new era was dawning in the treatment of infectious skin diseases and other internal ailments.[4] But in 1949 this was hardly public knowledge. It took many years before silica gel became recognized on the health food market.

Nature's Most Perfect Energizer

The biologically strengthening nature of silica can already be observed in the structure and support function of narrow, upright standing plants like horsetail.[5] By the year 1900, botanists could establish that silica also increases resistance to disease in plants by checking into the structural function of silica in living plant tissue.

---

* Dr. Becker's original formula colloidal mineral silica gel is produced by a well-reputed health food supplement manufacturer in Germany. It is officially approved by the very strict "neuform" health food standards. The German brand "Original Silicea Balsam" is available in Canada. In the USA the product is registered as the separate trademark "Body Essential Silica Gel." Despite the differences in name, the two products are identical in content. Both are colloidal silica gel derived from mineral silica as described.

It soon became clear that plants and animals and even humans – that all life forms depend on a constant supply of silica for structural and metabolic needs. For instance, in birds, 70 percent of plumage is silica. This is notably in line with silica's general effect on the outer covering of living things and its attachments, such as feathers in birds or skin, nails and hair in humans. Silica, we quickly discovered, is nature's building block. Then it was found to be even more than fundamental to life's structural maintenance. It was found, if I am permitted to paraphrase the words of the Kena Upanishad, "to first drive life to start on its journey."

Silica's Life Creation on Earth
The most logical and widely accepted scientific view of the creation of life on our planet comes from Nobel laureate Professor Butenandt. His explanations of creation draws on experiments that researchers Birkhofer and Ritter carried out about 1958. Butenandt's creation theory was confirmed by the Russian silica researcher Woronkow. This creation theory holds that silicon attaches temporarily to nitrogen and then splits after the formation of bodies that have the properties of albumen. Thus, in forming living albumin protein, it plays a significant role in the formation of life.

Life on earth, according to latest scientific findings, arose from electrical discharges in the prototype nitrogen and carbon atmosphere. These electrical discharges accumulated on silica dissolved in the primeval sea. This in turn caused the elementary building blocks of life, the amino acids.

At this early point in creation, the amino acids polymerized into albuminous, protein-like bodies. To show how this orig-ination theory is confirmed by the massive occurrence of silica armors of diatoms, we must sidetrack a little. So come along with me to the ocean.

Useful Dead or Alive

"Diatom" is the name given to any of over 5,000 species of algae of the class *Bacillariophyceae*. Diatoms are usually single-celled. Yet, occasionally they aggregate into small colonies by virtue of their sticky, gelatinous coating. Though also present in aerial and terrestrial environments, their main habitat is aquatic. They live in both freshwater and marine water. In the waters of earth they occupy mainly the top 100 meters, where sunlight is abundantly available.

These organisms are photosynthetic. They use fats and volutin,* not starches, as their food reserves. Diatoms form the main component of plankton, the primary food source for most aquatic creatures. So they form the very beginning of the marine-life food chain. They have other uses in death.

When diatoms die, their silica-rich cell walls remain behind and accumulate on the ocean floor in continuous layers that can be up to 3,000 feet thick. These siliceous remains, most abundant in the western part of the North American continent, are diatomaceous earth or diatomite. Their chalky deposit is useful in industrial filtering out of impurities, as an adsorbent, and as an insulator. You see, here is the essence of that foot powder again that stimulated my mineral silica research.

Let us return to life because besides serving in death, diatoms have a far more important meaning for life's continuous evolution. They supply 70 percent of the oxygen on our planet. All other plants contribute a mere 30 percent to the earth's oxygen mantle.

Through the decay of diatoms, because of the polymerization of silica in diatom skeletons, oxygen was first released into

---

* Denotes a basophilic substance, thought to be a nucleic acid, that occurs as granules in algae and similar life forms.

the atmosphere and started life on its splendid journey. Only after this process of decay could the utilization of oxygen begin (with the help of special enzymes). This process produced 32 times the amount of energy compared with that from fermentation of simple organisms, making the development of life possible.

Without silica, all life processes would slow down their metabolism after a short time. Protein synthesis would grind to a halt. Fat metabolism would increase. Cells would fatten. This is analogous to the fattening of cancer cells because of oxygen utilization disturbance, i.e., oxygen starvation. Does this mean silica plays a role in cancer therapy? You bet.

Diatom photosynthesis or the assimilation of diatoms would be inhibited without light. Yet this does not happen. Diatoms give off silica that in turn begins the metabolic processes. By that it is fulfilling the task normally assumed by light. This points to the possibility that silica constitutes an emergency reserve during difficult times when certain stress situations occur. It seems that we have yet more to expect from silica, perhaps in the millennium just ahead.

Diluted silica solutions from the earth have an affinity for plant cell membranes. They react easily with protein, for instance with cotton fibers. The solution makes the cotton hair cells strongly absorptive and adsorptive. Higher plants form silica inclusions, such as the epidermis cells of campanula types, cyperacious plants and grasses. The stinging bristle tops of stinging nettle become impregnated or turn into silica (silicify) like the hooked hair of hops.

The silica-dependent creation is more than conjecture. It was confirmed by experiment. The metabolism of diatoms without silica slows down. Protein synthesis comes to a halt. Normally, photosynthesis would be inhibited in dark spaces, yet, diatoms give off silica that takes over the task of light. The siliceous process[6] that appears as a siliceous substance in fixed form is active in all surfaces of the waves of the sea. It is also active in the mountains, in the epidermis of plants, in human and animal skin, and in the surface of their organs and cells. This is a splendid example of the divine formation process from the dynamic of the infiniteness of the cosmos.

Sourcing Silica Stores

At this point you may wonder how you can assure an adequate intake of silica in your daily food. When I was a boy, my mother constantly served me porridge made of oats. I hated it. She said it was good for me. There are some obvious choices to be made. You can start eating porridge. You might increase your consumption of onions even at the risk of offending your neighbor's sensitive nostrils. Onions have the greatest silica content with 17 percent silica content found through analysis of onion ash. Next comes red beet with 11 percent.[7] Red beet is an excellent food to eat and has been found to inhibit carcinogenic processes also. Other good sources of silica are barley, millet, potatoes, corn, rye, and whole wheat. Try to eat them as cereals rather than as baked goods.

But is this enough? Though the soil is replete with silicates, most of it does not contain silica in bioavailable form. Food processing often removes original silica content. Milled flour contains only two percent of the silicon originally present. The remaining silica present in foods is not easily absorbed by the body. Much of it passes through but is not bioavailable to the system. Then again, you might hate to eat oats.

However, to help you prepare for silica-rich meals in your kitchen, the following comprehensive alphabetic nutrient table, expressed in milligrams per 100 grams (mg/100 g),[8] will help:

Apples	1.0	Oats	600.0
Apricots	1.0	Oranges	1.0
Asparagus	18.0	Parsley	13.0
Barley	230.0	Pears	2.0
Beans	2.0	Peas	2.0
Caraway	5.0	Plums	3.0
Carrots	5.0	Potatoes	200.0
Cauliflower	9.0	Pumpkin	7.0
Celery	4.0	Rape Seeds	16.0
Chanterelles	9.0	Red Currant	3.0
Cherries	1.0	Red Beets	21.0
Corn	19.0	Red Pepper	2.0
Gooseberries	3.0	Rye	17.0
Grapes	4.0	Spinach	4.0
Green Cabbage	2.0	Strawberries	6.0
Horseradish	13.0	Sunflowers	15.0
Lettuce	6.0	Topinambur	36.0
Millet	500.0	Whole Wheat	160.0

Remember though, much of today's silica-containing foods are grown in soils that are overburdened with artificial fertilizers. Apart from ruining the soil, imprudent industry has done us the bad turn of polluting the air. Years of DDT and other insecticide spraying have left their mark. It is hardly surprising then that silica deficiency is widespread despite the apparent universal abundance of silica in the soil.

To assure adequate silica intake, it might be a good idea to supplement your diet with silica from a clean and unpolluted source, especially because our organisms must have more antioxidants like silica to empower them in their battle against pollution. This makes supplementation with a fast-absorbing silica like silica gel a good idea even if you make silica-containing foods a regular part of your diet.

Herbal Silica

Concentrating your eating on organically grown, silica-rich foods will help, but is it enough? The growing occurrence of silica deficiencies shows otherwise. The daily diet usually lacks sufficient quantities of assimilable silica. There are several other silica sources available. Among the herbs, horsetail has exceptional quantities of silica. Hemp, nettle and bird grass also contain silica. Medicinal herbal plants contain a protein-bound silica in a colloidal form.[9] Researcher Moleschott reported already in the year 1852 that his colleague Struve found 97 percent silica in equisetum (horsetail) ash. Another researcher, Brock, found 83 percent in a lime-rich habitat. According to research by Lindemann, knotgrass polygonum contains 0.2 percent soluble and 40 percent total silica in the bud stage. In contrast, in its withering stage, knotgrass polygonum contains from 0.2 percent to 80 percent total silica.

The content of soluble silica utilizable through animal and human organisms is of singular importance. Findings of silica content,[10] each according to habitat show a content of:

2,200 - 5,400 mg/100 g in horsetail
2,680 mg/100 g in herb galeopsis (wood tooth)
210 - 840 mg/100 g in herb polygoni (knotgrass)

Soil Silica

The effect of medicinal soil refers specifically back to its silica content. This amounts to approximately 58 to 60 percent. Newer analyses have even shown up to 65 percent. This suggests that the silica content forms the major healing agent in medicinal healing soils, also called diatomaceous earths. And as we have found out, the unqualified term "silica" refers to the naturally occurring mineral that consists of silicon dioxide and is found in substantial portions of the earth's crust.

Silica in Animals

"There is no tissue without silica," said Hugo Schulz. This conclusion is supported by researcher Kobert. His students found silica in almost all human and animal tissue in ash analysis. Herbivores have the highest blood and tissue content of silica. Carnivores have the lowest amounts. Again, silica content depends upon dietary intake. Middle values are typical for humans who are omnivorous. The following values are very different according to method of determination (see above cautionary note). SiO_2 amounts in mg/100 g in animals:

Animal fetal tissue	Flaschen/Träger	Monceaux	Schweigart
calf, mouse	4.22		
liver			690
brain			410
muscle			330
blood: horse	1.2		
cattle		14	410
dog		0.55	
rabbit	14 - 32	1.26	
cow's milk	2.0 - 2.5		

The above values should be taken with a "grain of silica." Earlier data on the distribution of silicon in animal tissues have varied greatly because of the measuring problem with lab equipment made of glass. Modern studies are more accurate because they make use of plastic ware among other stricter precautions.

Non-Toxicity in Mice

Toxicity tests done with colloidal silica gel in 1980 on healthy lab mice under regular conditions for 14 days showed that the gel is practically non-toxic even at high concentrations. Test dosages were increased from 10 ml/kg to 40 ml/kg without the animals showing any incompatibility whatsoever. This shows that the absolute minimal dosage that could possibly be lethal would have to be far in excess of 40 ml/kg. Such values are not likely to be reached under general conditions. Colloidal silica gel contains 2.8 g of silicic acid per 100 ml.[11]

Silica in Humans
In human blood there are three forms of silica: 10 percent is water soluble silica, 60 percent binds to albumin bodies, and 30 percent binds to fats. Silica loss in humans differs according to individual metabolism and nutritional habits. It averages about 10 to 40 mg per 24 hour period. Substantial ongoing silica elimination occurs via the urine and the intestines with additional loss coming from skin scaling, hair, and nail cuttings. This constantly ongoing and unavoidable silica loss must be factored into a meaningful silica food and supplementation program.

	Flaschen/Träger	Monceaux	Schweigart
Human ash			
nails	16	360	
blood		2.4	
mother's milk		0.72	
thymus gland			310
suprarenal capsule		250	
pancreas			30
heart			8
liver	9.0		8.7
kidney			6.1
brain			5.6
small intestine		4.6	
thymus		16.2	
fibrin		30.0	
lens		0.2	

Silicon in human tissue	in humans	in dry tissue
goiter	43	
lungs	1200	90-40
lymph glands	1,200	
nails	360	
spleen	520	28
tendons	6	
thyroid gland	8	
umbilical cord	25 – 40	

The elimination of silica with urine in mg/100 cm^3 amounts in:

dogs	0.9 - 1.5
sheep	12 - 17
cats	0.5 - 0.7
guinea pigs	14 - 28
rabbits	11 - 2.7
rats	3 - 5

Despite the variances, it can be seen that silica, established in the ash of embryonic or very young tissue, is mostly higher than in older tissue. The amount of silica found is chiefly dependent upon the amount of connective tissue found in the tested organs. This makes much sense because human connective tissue is richest in silica.

Silica's Biological Synthesis

While silica in a finely dispersed colloidal form predominates in the body of youngsters and contributes greatly to their greater bounce and flexibility, the inactive form is mainly stored in the organisms of older individuals in hair and nails. We can conclude from this that there is an ongoing silica metabolism in special need of support in aging individuals.

The important tissue task of silica can be helped once the increasing loss of silica content is apparent in the body. Silica loss occurs simultaneously with colloidal physical tissue change, specifically connective tissue. With the ingestion of supplementary silica gel, cell metabolism can be reactivated. The cell's ability for division, i.e., duplication and new growth, can be stimulated.

The tissue aging process can be reversibly affected. Newly silica-enriched, cell tissue can again function as a rejuvenating biocatalyst that stimulates metabolism. Genuine reversal of aging symptoms (in contrast to the mere slowing down of the aging process) is something entirely new to gerontology. We will take a closer look at this exciting research.

Important knowledge of the effects of silica come from experiments[12] with diatom cyclotella. The formation of chrysosis (leucosin) stopped in a silica-free nutrient solution after 12 to 14 hours. The synthesis of carotenoid stopped after nine hours. It also choked photosynthetic O_2 production. After six to eight hours RNA, chlorophyll, and total protein synthesis was almost completely blocked.

Glutamic acid decrease and a decrease in the pools of alpha ketoglutamic acid, from the primary material of protein formation, precedes the inhibition of protein synthesis. In contrast, fat; i.e., fatty acid synthesis, increases by 100 percent. These findings show that silica metabolism is closely and specifically related with other syntheses and that silica plays a far more important role than just as a cell wall stabilizer.

Practicing Prevention
It is said that practicing prevention is an expensive, time-consuming and useless effort. Government publications and certain medical circles tell us not to supplement our diets with vitamins and minerals. "After all," the argument goes, "you cannot know what you may be preventing." Nothing could be further from the truth. I have been practicing prevention for the last 30 years, at considerable expense, I might add.

It is true, I did not always exactly know what I was preventing. I just wanted to make sure that I did not contract a chronic ailment or disease that would incapacitate me, cripple me or leave me in persistent pain. I can happily report to you that my personal prevention program, which includes dietary and supplementary means, works for me. I am over 50 and in perfect health. I have never been ill, never had to be in the hospital, never had to be operated on. To me, that is prevention and it works.

The key to fighting essential silica loss lies in continuous fortification, starting as early as possible. Treating silica supplements like an old age pension plan that you start at age 20 for reimbursement at age 65 promises the best long term prevention. Because even without noticeable silica deficiency symptoms, such as dry, wrinkled skin, dull, lifeless hair and brittle nails, prevention should be practised. You may not know what you are preventing now, but if you are still full of bounce at age 100, you may have an inkling of what you prevented. Are you ready to entrust your longevity to your government?

Turning Back the Aging Clock with Vitamin C and Silica Gel
Evidence of another vital supplement, vitamin C, will show why long term supplementation is the best prevention. In 1992 the news reported that Linus Pauling, the famous and health-wise double Nobel laureate,[*] underwent treatment for prostate cancer. Reporters made the most of Pauling's succumbing to this cancer despite his enormous intake of 300 times the recommended daily requirement of vitamin C.

Pauling claims that vitamin C helps to prevent cancer. Accordingly, he ingested vitamin C at the fearful rate of 18,000 mg daily, faithfully for over 25 years. "So," you say, "we can conclude from this that despite his immense pre-

[*] 1954 Nobel Prize for Chemistry for his work with vitamin C; 1962 Noble Peace Prize.

43

vention program he contracted cancer and that long term vitamin C supplementation is useless."

In 1992, Linus Pauling completed 91 years on earth. In view of this, his personal supplementation program remains immensely impressive. He beat the average life expectancy for North American males by a whopping twenty years. And he did even better than that. His doctors reported very good response to cancer therapy at the time this was written. Pauling's immune system responded so well to treatment that his prostate cancer was considered healed.

You might find it remarkable that the enzyme that is prerequisite in the body to form collagen (a precondition for the successful formation of most bones) must contain vitamin C. In the absence of vitamin C, the enzyme becomes dysfunctional. This dysfunction was a familiar problem to British sailors before the advent of the late 18th century. On long journeys they developed scurvy due to vitamin C deficiency in their dry rations. On the suggestion of James Lynd, limes were added to their rations. British sailors were nicknamed "limeys," but henceforth didn't get scurvy. Turn to the subheading "The Silicon Factor" to find out more about the important connection of silicon and the enzyme for making collagen.

Colloidal Aging

If that was a plug for vitamin C or indirectly for carbon, there is even more convincing evidence of the anti-aging, anti-degenerative, rejuvenating significance of silica in the human colloidal system, specifically in the connective tissue. All the vitamin C in the world is not going to stimulate the growth of connective tissue if silica is not present in sufficient quantities.[*]

Human tissue, of course, is a complex system of colloids.[13] The colloids occur on the boundary surfaces of the inner tissue. Every colloid (including out-of-body silica gel) has the

---

[*] Of course, silicon needs vitamin C for enzymatic activity.

tendency to enlarge its particles with progressive aging. What that means is that it splits off water (a process called syneresis) and by that diminishes its available reactive surface.

Tissue swelling is of greatest significance for the biological functioning of protein structures, especially the collagen fibre of connective tissue and muscle fibre. Through swelling, several hundred percent of the protein weight of water can be absorbed. Polar-constructed hydrotropic material such as urea, thiourea, and especially silica, promotes this type of desirable swelling.

In 1959, excited by the colloid chemical views of researcher M. H. Fischer, O. Scholl and K. Letters examined the influence of soluble lower molecular silica on protein's water-binding ability. In a series of experiments, a standard-base-protein-acid mixture was suffused with hydrochloric acid. Saturation of a sodium caseinate containing 67 percent water continued until 70 percent hydrochloric acid was obtained.

Already in 1935, researcher W. Moninger stabilized protein-containing foam with small amounts of silica sol. This is due to the enclosing film of water between the two mono-molecular protein layers. The water is binding with protein in a swelling. This prevents the water from discharging and therefore improves stability. The silica effect, according to Moninger, "comes from the positively charged protein's ability to react with the negatively charged silica sol during discharging and dispersion increase." This is known as the "opalescence phenomenon."

Aged skin is therefore favorably influenced by silica. Researcher Saller confirmed that: the younger the individual, the higher the silica content in the organism. Saller ascribes a healing power to silica preparations and drugs for aging phenomena. Low molecular silica of one percent colloidal form[14] stabilizes the water-combining ability.

Accordingly, prevention of premature aging to some degree depends upon augmenting the water-protein combination. In the aging process, the protein in living tissue "unswells" and the surfaces shrink. This leads to a cessation of enzyme reactions. As particles enlarge, less water is available. Therefore the process of tissue aging is primarily a colloid physical change of proteins. A reduction in the size of the "inner surface" occurs. It is, however, the inner cell surface or boundary area that forms the basis for the life processes.

Diminishing the inner surface in size limits and inhibits it. The primary process of natural aging is of such typical colloidal processes. It is dehydration of cell protein in flocculation (a kind of clumping) and coagulation phenomena. These in turn cause altered diffusion and osmosis of membranes. Does this not all remind you of the colloidal swelling that occurs in silica gel formations? Can silica gel reverse this aging process? I think, yes, it can.

It was determined that with aging phenomena an increase in the blood silica content resulted from one percent colloidal silica and a "making young" of the vascular wall protein in arteriosclerosis. Blood pressure went down, lymphocytes and phagocytes could be significantly increased.[15] These findings confirm that silica gel boosts the human immune system.

In related animal experiments, a strong increase in the number of lymphocytes and phagocytes was also produced according to J. Mezger. Both of these cell categories must be recognized as having the most important relationship with lymph glands. Therefore silica is a good remedy with lymphatic diathesis and tuberculosis of the lymph glands of the neck as well.

With early and late scrofula increased salivation occurs frequently. In affected adults, salivation usually occurs during sleep and is detectable by a moist pillow. In affected children this is often observed as "slobbering." The moist pillow is also attributable to the parallel occurrence of head perspiration in children. Silica addresses this well, according to researcher Hermann Hädeler. The additional prescribing of calcium phosphate is necessary since bone and gland growth and development disorders play a role with children.

The New Science of "Youthening"
Man's absolute maximum life span always has been the same at around 120 years. The recently discovered mummified body of an ancient Austrian shepherd found in the Alps near the Italian border showed an amazingly well preserved corpse. It revealed a body well advanced in years but still featuring a good set of teeth. It seems he died accidentally. This anthropological health record of an ancient shepherd of perhaps 40 years of age contrasts sharply with average longevity of his day. In the caves at the dawn of human history it was a brief span of 20 years, perhaps due to unsanitary conditions and the ravages of frequent tribal wars.

Over the millennia that hardly improved because even with the advent of nations, high infant mortality and infectious diseases were killing off people in their prime. In the days of the Roman Empire, reaching 22 years of age still was considered lucky for similar reasons. Even as recently as around 1900 AD, people were old at age 40.

Yet today, longevity in the West is somewhere between 75 to 80 years. It is constantly climbing because of prevention practice, dietary supplementation and medical advances. We also tend to live longer if we are less afraid of becoming old. Having children later in life also tends to increase maximum longevity. If current trends continue, people will be reaching an average of 85 years by the year 2000 due to optimal nutrition and exercise. Some projections see us reaching 100 before long. Others are even more optimistic.

While the phenomenon of aging once was considered beyond human understanding, there now appears a startling simplicity. Aging seems to be regulated by our genes over which science is achieving ever greater control. So, for the most part, aging is now becoming reversible. Gerontology, the science of "youthening" as I call it, claims startling new successes. Tremendous increases in longevity – doubling the normal life span – are produced in animals when their food intake is sharply restricted. Dietary controls seem to enhance the body's anti-aging chemistry.

There's much talk of the human growth hormone DHEA (short for dehydroepiandrosterone) that apparently reverses the effects of aging and is currently being tested. Apparently, aging sets in when the body becomes slowly depleted of this hormone starting after the age of 30. At 50, most people secrete only 30 percent of what they produced when they were young. This loss can cause great health deterioration. Early test results with DHEA injections into older people have been surprisingly successful, but there may be unwanted side effects, as is often the case with hormonal treatments.

A most unwanted "side effect" of increasing longevity itself is that geriatric diseases are ever more threatening to an aging population. So we are promised to grow older, but we cannot retain the "baby bounce" and zest of youth that makes life worth living. So what good is it all? What about the increase in degenerative diseases? Can they be stopped? This is going to be gerontology's greatest hurdle, but help is on the way with the premise that aging is not in itself a disease, but that it just makes the body more vulnerable to disease. Silica, the stuff babies have in abundance, can give the body elasticity into old age. You may have enough bounce left to really jump for joy as you reach age 100. It is known that silica content in living tissue is at its highest during the embryonic stages.[16] This points to a possible rejuvenating effect of silica gel. To find out if this may be so, we will now turn to plasma protein and its reactions and relationships.

Aiding the Body's Water-Binding Ability

Plasma proteins can combine with acids and with bases, a capability labeled "amphoteric." Plasma proteins that are forming large supermolecules, are albumin bodies. They are colloidal proteins built up mainly of amino acids. Albumins are heat coagulable and are soluble in water.

Albumin bodies, like egg white, blood plasma, and milk, can absorb great amounts of water in their binding. This gives them the ability to expand. Albumins make up about half the total proteins in the blood plasma and play a major role in maintaining proper distribution of fluid between the blood and the tissues. This ability to maintain fluid balance is crucial to the body. When the level of albumins in the blood drops (which happens in long term starvation)* the tissues retain water and a condition called edema results.

This means that the most important precondition for the biological processes occurring in cell plasma is the ability to optimize water combination and the resultant swelling of albumin bodies. The relationship of acids to bases within the proteins influence this swelling ability. How can it be stimulated or amplified?

---

* Starvation must not be confused with fasting. Starvation is debilitating. Fasting, especially juice fasting, is cleansing and invigorating. I wrote the book, *The Joy of Juice Fasting,* for a guide to fasting for rejuvenation, cleansing and weight loss.

The most favorable combination with water in albumin proteins is reached at a sodium chloride content of 0.9 percent. The albumins' maximum swelling ability results from the addition of not more than 70 percent of hydrochloric acid. The hydrochloric acid is necessary to neutralize the alkaline condition of the protein. In this way more than 400 percent water can be combined as hydration water. In this condition the colloidal albumin dissolves water-insoluble fats, lipoids (cholesterol), and esters.

The hydrating or water-binding ability of cytoplasmic substance is controlled through a balanced acid-base-albumin relationship. It is of fundamental importance to the elementary life processes in cells. The breaking down, the building up and the enzyme reactions in cell metabolism can proceed at peak capacity only in highly hydrated protein.

As the body ages, the accumulations of poisons, bacteria, toxins and carcinogens finally lead to a disturbance of the albumin protein's water-binding ability. This, in turn, leads to a structural disintegration with all resultant phenomena of shrinkage. In living tissue this occurs as coagulation, hardening and blood pressure increase. These are familiar aging symptoms. Before we can reach for the right "gun" to fight it off, we need to take a closer look at the biochemistry involved.

A protein molecule in solution has a three-dimensional globular structure. Proteins are made up of chains of amino acids. These amino acids fall into two categories, hydrophillic (water attracting) and hydrophobic (water repelling). Hydrophillic residues tend to be found near the surface of the molecule, facing the solvent (water). Hydrophobic residues are normally found towards the interior of the molecule, away from the solvent (water). The hydrophillic affinity for swelling is greatly helped by the presence of polar constructed hydrotrophic silica, which promotes swelling, thereby preventing shrinkage, coagulation and hardening of tissues.

Chapter Four

The soul of man
Resembles water:
From heaven it comes,
To heaven it rises,
And again below,
To the earth it goes,
Forever fluid...
...Human soul
How like water you are!

*Goethe**

The Great Discovery –
The Pristine Waters of Fiji

Without water there is no life. Water is the essence and the medium of life. It is the mysterious source that spawns creation and sustains it. The living body's ceaseless moisture-seeking and water retention endeavors are greatly assisted by silica's positive hydrotropism, which bestows the ability to fix water in place. Just how vital silica's water-binding ability is can be gleaned from the fact that our bodies consist of 70 percent water. Water is required in abundance for flushing toxins. It is a clinical fact that poor hydration dramatically increases the risk of disease. This is why I counsel to drink six to eight glasses of water daily. But by that advice a dilemma arises. Which water is still fit to drink?

* Translated from the German by Klaus Kaufmann.

The Princeton Problem

Cumulative water pollution, caused by a multitude of agricultural, industrial, human, and animal waste has made much of our drinking water undrinkable. This is true also of waters in the less populous regions of the advanced nations. One of the worst examples is occurring even now at my doorstep in British Columbia, Canada. On January 16, 1997, the region of Princeton, BC, prohibited the use of tap water for drinking because viral contamination caused serious illness. All tap water must be boiled. Bottled water quickly sold out, and had to be imported. The hospital began cooking using only bottled water, not trusting even the boiling of tap water to be sufficient protection.

When interviewed, the mayor of Princeton reassured the public. The city was adding chlorine to the municipal water supply, thereby 'overcoming the problem in a couple of weeks and making the water safe again for drinking.' Really? In my book, chlorine is very poisonous and highly irritating to the mucous membranes. Yes, it can kill germs even in greatly diluted concentrations in water. This makes chlorine popular for making water "safe." Personally, I stay far away even from swimming pools treated with chlorine because it burns my eyes, let alone entertaining the thought of drinking such chlorinated water.

To avoid drinking water treated with chlorine or alum, the obvious choice is finding or creating sources of pure water and drinking only that instead of tap water. Taking it either directly from the source or if that is not possible, using good bottled water that comes from a truly natural, unpolluted spring nearby —if there is one—is great. But what do you drink when there is no spring and groundwater is scarce? The person who said, "Water, water everywhere—but not a drop to drink," meant that huge salty brine, the ocean, where indeed potable water is as difficult to come by as it is today in Princeton, BC.

Wakaya

Some forty years ago, a conference took place in Toronto, Ontario, Canada. In a brainstorming session, executives met to ascertain macroeconomics regions of the future. They focused their projection on the yet impossibly far away turn of the century, the new millennium, the year 2000! Existing macroeconomics were then running mainly vertical—north to south. Most group members also identified Germany as the major economic power in the future Europe. Yet one of the executives, then the president of Volvo, suggested that the Pacific Rim would be the hub of future macroeconomics. He delineated the Pacific ring as made up of New Zealand, Australia, Indonesia, Singapore, Malaysia, China, Japan, Canada, the USA, Mexico, Peru, and Chile. Then he added, "the very center of this ring deep in the Pacific Ocean is Fiji. It will become the gateway to the Pacific." A young man by the name of David Harrison Gilmour attended this meeting. David decided to check out what this fellow from Volvo was talking about. David went to Fiji. He immediately marveled at its great beauty and treasured its unsullied beaches and charming people.

Even back then David saw that Fiji would be safe from pollution, pesticides, and acid rain because it is located some 2,400 km (1,500 miles) from the nearest continent and has no polluting industry. David Gilmour, who was consulting me on silica, said, "I fell in love with the people and the place. Even today, the 332 islands of the Republic of Fiji comprise the last bastion of ecological sanctity in our world." Then David told me of another fascination that had followed him throughout his life: WATER!

David's mother was an opera singer; his father was a renowned athlete and merchant banker. Not surprisingly, much of David's childhood was spent traveling the world, getting to know waters everywhere. In 1937, at the age of seven, David was with his parents in the water-treatment spa of Baden-Baden, Germany, famous for its silica-rich healing waters. Water made a lasting impression on him.

Potable water represents a mere 1% of the 70% of the planet's water. A precisian at heart, David Gilmour was always on the lookout for a source of pure and healthy water. Says he, "Even many bottled waters are far from exciting when you check out the source." In Fiji, David made a discovery that fulfilled a boyhood dream: owning a Pacific island! "When I found the island of Wakaya, I envisioned this uninhabited island to be developed with a touch of style and integrity," David reveals.

Wakaya is an unspoiled island of breathtaking beauty. The island has 600 foot elevations and 32 white sand beaches. Hundreds of fallow deer, wild horses, and boar roam Wakaya today. Broad expanses of flat land bracket the northern and southern tips. Over the next 20 years David Gilmour and his wife Jill created on Wakaya a very special island home for themselves and for their friends. Nature was munificent in creating Wakaya a unique 2,200-acre gem.

David acquired Wakaya in 1972. He bemoaned the commercialization of many of the world's exotic destinations. He wanted to make sure that this could never happen to Wakaya. In 1991, David and Jill decided to share Wakaya by building an exquisite and enchanting world class resort that has since become the smallest deluxe resort in the world. This was accomplished with the help of Robert and Lynda Miller, now the managers of the island resort, and J. Jay Boland, who has taken on the task of spreading the good word around about Wakaya from their Los Angeles office. By the way, Lynda Miller is an ardent Kombucha drinker!

The Gilmours and their friends also created a beautiful village for the Fijians who maintain the island. The village includes a small 19th century-style church plus a nostalgic schoolhouse. Naming the new resort the Wakaya Club, the Gilmours made their island home into a holiday retreat of the highest integrity. There are many diversions. Holiday activities include golf, scuba diving, tennis, hiking, deep-sea fishing and many more. But growth on Wakaya is carefully controlled. The island facilities will not be expanded to any great degree.

So, if it's luxurious privacy you want, Wakaya offers it together with discretion. The Wakaya Club accommodates only twelve couples at any one time! Today Wakaya is one of the world's top ten luxury resorts. Says Gilmour, "To extend our vision of paradise, we set out to identify a source of pure natural bottled water for our guests. As a result, in 1992 we invested in a small water bottling business on the island of Viti Levu, the main island of Fiji."

Water of Viti
Have you ever wondered why natural springs bubble forth forever? Where does that endless flow of water come from? The secret is rainfall, which ultimately feeds all natural springs and underground water reservoirs. Some of this rainfall flows into the oceans by forming rivulets, then streams and rivers. Some of it is used up right away by flora and fauna. Some of it disappears into the bowels of the earth. Some of the water can remain hidden for decades or longer in underground water reservoirs.

The healthiest water we can drink is rainwater from an unpolluted atmosphere. The amount of rainfall is determined by the proportion of water and land. So it is not surprising to find the greatest amount of rainfall in and around the Pacific basin, the world's greatest body of water that covers nearly one half of the globe. The warming rays of the sun turn the uncontaminated waters of Viti into vapor that is lifted out of the ocean, free from salt, carried into the sky and deposited as pristine rain water on the higher elevations, the mountainous region. As the clouds pass over the peaks of the volcanic Nakauvadra Mountains of Viti Levu, the colder mountain air cools the clouds and in a gradual cooling process turns the vapor into condensation of moisture in the gentlest of rain.

Aquifer

Janusz Kubs, David's partner in the water venture, drove through the Nakauvadra Mountains in search of water. His curiosity was triggered when he observed a Japanese hydro-geology team conducting tests in the area. Janusz decided to do his own testing. To his great delight he found a vast store of underground water 200 feet below the surface in the Yaqara Range of the Nakauvadra Mountains.

This water, he found, filters through a water-bearing formation of fragmented basalt rock, sandstone and other natural silicates within a 15 km diameter volcanic crater going back to the early tertiary period, i.e., about 4-5 million years ago, into an aquifer deep beneath volcanic highlands and pristine tropical forests. The water permeates at an extremely slow rate through the strata, taking several decades to reach the underground crater. This implied that the water would be low in bicarbonates. Surprise, surprise, lab testing for trace elements revealed also an amazingly high amount of silica. David and Janusz asked themselves, "Silica? What will this do to us?" It intrigued them. They did some searching and eventually came across my books on the topic.

Doug Carlson, a friend and associate of David's who lives not too far from Vancouver, contacted me. Before I knew it, I found myself flying to Fiji to check out the colloidal silica in this water and explain the uses during a plant opening ceremony. You can well imagine the joy that was spread throughout the island nation when it became suddenly clear that Fiji Pure Natural Water contained the hitherto most overlooked, most important mineral in almost identical proportion to the famous Dunaris well, that is, 81 mg/l.

Thorough and repeated lab testing showed Fiji Pure Natural Water to contain the healthiest form of silica, precipitated in natural rainwater from a pollution-free atmosphere. In a fortuitous stroke of fate, I was privileged to discover the world's most unique source of precipitated silica suspended in readily absorbable colloidal form. The real boon was to find this silica-rich drinking water in a region free of polluting industry, far from acid rain, nuclear power stations, atomic testing, pesticides, detergents, and other carcinogens that plague so many regions of our planet.

Geological tests show that the aquifer can provide up to one million liters of pure drinking water daily. What makes it unique is its naturally high level of silica - several times higher than in any other drinking water available today. I found that in addition to being an excellent source of colloidal silica, the water contains traces of other minerals. Its total mineral composition in mg/l turned out to be in alphabetical order:

Bicarbonates	140
Calcium (Ca)	16
Chloride (Cl)	5.4
Magnesium (Mg)	13
Potassium (K)	4
Silica (SiO2)	81
Sodium	18
Sulfate, as SO4	0.6

This water has a very low sodium content and is very low in bicarbonates as well. With a count of 7.2, the water also has a neutral pH. Total dissolved solids amount to 160 PPM (mg/l). Other minerals are, as expected, present in negligible trace quantities below 1 mg/l. As shown above, the water has a very low calcium and magnesium content. This gives it a *supersoft* and refreshing taste. In fact, the great taste—with no aftertaste—was one of the first things I noticed. A disturbing aftertaste usually comes from a high magnesium and calcium content. After all, who needs calcium and magnesium when you have got plenty of silica (see Chapter Nine)? Perhaps I found it the most remarkable that the mercury count (Hg) came to only <0.00005 mg/l. This is one of the best indicators for the pristine conditions of the underground environment in which this water accumulates.

In the words of David Gilmour, "I appreciated your good news all the more because I was close to another Canadian, Dr. Shute, who discovered vitamin E. That too was not understood for years. Medical doctors were generally totally resentful of preventive medicine. I suffered from ischemia at the time. Had I not taken vitamin E for the last twenty years, I would have died five years ago. Vitamin E supplementation gave me enough oxygen to avoid a heart attack. So I decided to invest a great deal of money in this water. Learning that the colloidal silica in the water may be even more important than vitamin E makes my investment a dream come true."

Then he continues, "As the saying goes, I have put my money and mind where my mouth is. I wanted to see it come true because there are ever increasingly educated, health conscious and active people to appreciate purity. The purity of this water was the reason for the search. With health the result, my dream of pure water has come true just as my dream of Wakaya has. The most ecology-conscious island backed by the most pristine water. This is a greater discovery than I dreamed possible."

A new venture for producing Fiji Pure Natural Water was the result. As could be expected from a virgin ecosystem, further testing showed this water to be indeed beautifully pure. No harmful contaminants of any kind can be found in Fiji or its pure natural water. It turns out that this water is acknowledged as the purest of all drinking waters in the world! Bottled at source from a relatively limitless supply, this pristine water full of colloidal silica is now shipped worldwide. Outside the Fijian nation the initial overseas consumers for this water are in California and in Japan.

Exploring Yaqara

I was, of course, at the plant opening. The President of Fiji, His Excellency, Ratu Sir Kamisese Mara opened the bottling plant on November 9, 1996, following traditional Fijian ceremonies. This included the preparation of the Yaqona, the traditional Fijian ceremonial drink. In his opening address, Ratu Mara told the more than 160 invited guests that, "Here is a company, which will prosper by sharing with the world our pristine natural water." The Fijian government granted the bottling company, Natural Waters of Viti Limited, a 99 years lease on the land.

The multimillion-dollar project is erected directly over the aquifer. After checking out bottling facilities around the world, the plant was designed and built according to state-of-the-art water filtering and bottling technology. The water of the aquifer is actually safe to drink straight from the source however; it undergoes filtering and ozonation processes to comply with international regulations. The water treatment operation precludes any possibility of human contact with the water during the bottling process.

A triple layer of protection includes filtration to 0.2 microns, ozonation of the filtered water in a completely closed system from the aquifer to the bottle. Then the bottle making operation and the bottling take place in a clean room purification system that provides particle-free and microorganism-free air and surfaces. Positive air pressure coupled with a state-of-the-art air filtering system keep the rooms clean and free of dust particles at all times.

High temperatures ensure sterile bottles. Computer automated filling systems minimize the need for human operators. Newly manufactured bottles are first rinsed with ozonated product water before being filled with fresh water. Fiji Pure Natural Water comes in 500 ml, 1 l, and 1.5 l award-winning design bottles that show a map of Fiji in relation to the world on the back of the bottle.

The bottles are of recyclable PET resin, one of the most environmentally beneficial packaging materials today. PET resin does not create waste. It is recycled into fabrics used in outdoor apparel, such as skiwear. The ecofriendly raw material for PET resin is purified terophthalic acid (PTA). The leaching of estrogen-like compounds from certain hydrocarbons and plastics that reportedly create dangerous hormone imbalances comes from other types of plastic that contain nonylphenol. This is not in PET so that this bottling method is by far the safest.

Bottling itself proceeds according to strict hygiene requirements that conform to the Food Standards Code of Australia as well as the Food and Drug Administration of the United States. The filled and capped bottles are date stamped and safety sealed. The Yaqara plant can provide up to one million liters of water a day, thus has a total capacity of 360 million liters per year. However, initial production is being limited to 25 million liters per year.

The plant has recently achieved the highest honor, that of International Standards Organization's quality assurance program certification, a certificate of worldwide validity (ISO9002:1994).

After the opening ceremony I took out time to explore the Yaqara Range. I had an extensive talk with the plant's geologist. It struck me what a wonderful idea it would be to open a health spa at Yaqara. The beautiful, rugged terrain of the Yaqara Mountain Range on the Island of Viti Levu is a perfect spot for a silica spa for regeneration and healing. The silica-rich, Fiji Pure Natural Water, once bottled, is only for drinking. It is far too dear for bathing in it. Yet bathing in silica is extremely beneficial to the skin. Still, I will have to wait until my Spa at Yaqara can become a reality. At least I already have an expert hydrotherapist greatly interested in running such a health spa.

Meanwhile, this "Water of Viti" is ready and already a hot tourist item in the gift shops of the Fijian tourist spots. I am writing this sitting back here in Vancouver at my computer and drinking my eight glasses of Fiji Pure Natural Water a day. Each time I quench my thirst with this best of all drinking waters, I take in the most beneficial colloidal silica. It sure helps to keep these "old bones" rejuvenated!

Chapter Five

"The sagacious reader who is capable of reading
between the lines that which does not stand
written in them, but is nevertheless implied, will
be able to form some conception."
Johann Wolfgang von Goethe, Poet (1749-1832)

Curative Cultured Crystals

External Healing from Head to Toe
The focus of health concern has improved. "Fix me quickly,
doctor" has been replaced with "How can I prevent it?" A
good example is the fact that, for heart disease, modern
medicine now recognizes the disease-preventing value of
regularly eating nuts, as practised by "health nuts" Seventh
Day Adventists for many years.

After unsuccessfully trying to "cure" degenerative disease
with drug therapy, side effects much worse than those
caused by immunization are increasingly driving us to find
better ways of healing. The best therapy is the nutritional
approach. Nutrition is today's medicine, both as a curative
remedy and as a preventive aspect of lifestyle. We must
learn time and again that our food must be our medicine
and our medicine should be contained in our food.

Beginning in the Mouth
Silica gel is the remedy of choice with diseases in the upper
body regions. These include tonsillitis, gum disease, pharynx
or air canal catarrh,[17] enlarged throat lymph glands, ozena,
chronic pharyngitis and laryngitis, paranasal sinus suppurations, mastoiditis, colds, middle ear catarrh and osteosclerosis.

The upper respiratory tract responds well to the use of silica gel. A good way to apply it is as a mouthwash, and then taking it internally to supplement the effectiveness. Rinsing with silica gel is good for laryngitis. Because of the beneficial effect on the lymphatic system, silica gel can help reduce swelling of the lymph nodes in the throat. The intake of silica also acts as a supportive treatment for inflammation of the middle ear.

Toughening the Teeth
Rinsing with silica gel is therapeutic in cases of gingivitis or ulitis, bleeding gums and tooth cavities. By hardening the enamel, silica gel assists to prevent cavities and preserve teeth. It also helps to prevent gum recession. The best success for gum recession can be obtained with a toothpaste produced from a silica base, according to research done by Kober. He reported a clear improvement of gum inflammation with 43 patients after four to five days. Cavities also improved. If you cannot find a silica tooth paste, simply brush your teeth and gums with silica gel on a daily basis to strengthen teeth and gums. Put some silica gel on your regular tooth brush and then brush gently.

Swirling diluted silica gel in your mouth for several minutes is also effective. For this purpose and for gargling and rinsing take two tablespoons of silica gel and dilute them with two ounces of lukewarm water. Then rinse or gargle for at least one minute. Spit out, but do not rinse with clear water so that some silica gel remains.

Respiratory Respite
The elasticity of lung tissue and its functioning depends on silica. Therefore, as a base therapy for lung and respiratory tract disorders, silica gel is indispensable. It is often prescribed in Europe because it simultaneously strengthens the immune system. Silica is especially important for pulmonary

tuberculosis. If silica joins the medication prescribed by the doctor, then tuberculosis germs in the lungs isolate faster.

Silica gel can supplement more orthodox therapy for lung disease. With bronchitis, silica gel acts as an anti-inflammatory. It promotes mucous flow and reduces coughing. Similarly breathing organs, coughing, and expectoration improve and heal through regeneration of mucous membranes.

Treating Tuberculosis

An old folk remedy in Russia is a silica-rich diet of whole grain millet purée fed to tuberculosis victims. Researcher Kobert and Gonnerman found that 20 g of dry millet seed contain nearly 100 mg of soluble silicon compounds! Silica is the specific agent for tuberculosis. It stimulates the inter-stitial tissue to fibrous induration and to encapsulation of the tuberculous focus.

Not so long ago, medicine had concluded that tuberculosis was conquered. This is unfortunately not true. It just reced-ed for a time. In the USA, in 1992, tuberculosis was on the rise. Atlanta, GA recorded a 50 percent increase of cases. Other cities across the USA like Newark, New Jersey and New York did not lag far behind. The increase is attributed partially to the rise in AIDS and partially to poverty and a concomitant lack of proper hygiene.

I would add poor nutrition! This seems borne out by the fact that ever more children under the age of five succumb to tuberculosis. Many healthy people, with strong immune defense, though carriers of the bacillus, never contract the disease. These circumstances point to an urgent need for a focused nutritional therapy.

Silica gel is a highly specific remedy in tuberculosis where an actual silica deficiency exists, specifically 50 percent.[18]

Researcher A. Charnot found a lower amount of silica in tuberculosis-predisposed guinea pigs than in receptive animals such as squirrels and goats. In addition, there is an almost complete lack of silica in the bones of tuberculosis patients.

A large silica deficiency exists in the lung tissues of tuberculosis sufferers. Silica storage diminishes and the connective tissue of the lung loses resistance to the tissue fusing caused by tubercle bacilli.[19] Energetic silica therapy results in stimulation of the interstitial connective tissue. This leads to fibrous induration and tissue increase and ultimately leads to the encapsulation of the focus.

"Silicafying" therapy for lung tuberculosis goes back to Schulz and Kobert, who recommended the therapy in 1917. The stricken lung area finally gains power to form new connective tissue and to heal the tissue areas that had deteriorated. This has been accepted by researchers B. von Kühn and Baumeister who arrived at the same or similar formula.

Digestive Disorders and Intestinal Illnesses
Silica gel is advantageous for the treatment of kidney and bladder disorders and inflammations and can prevent kidney stones. Silica increases urination up to 37 percent. Because of its anti-inflammatory, disinfecting and absorbing effects, silica gel acts to relieve gastrointestinal catarrh, ulcers caused by bacteria, bloating, and sometimes even constipation and hemorrhoids.

Applying silica gel compresses to hemorrhoidal tissue will accelerate the healing process. Treatment should continue overnight. Gastroenteral illnesses, such as dyspepsia, flatulence, diarrhea, enteritis, colitis, duodenal ulcers responded favorably to silica therapy. Constipation cleared up.

In his 1948 work on abdominal typhus and colloidal silica, W. Ruge states in the *Swiss Medical Weekly* that "already with healthy people colloidal silica functions as exceptionally appetite stimulating and leads to leucocytosis. Both effects depend upon activation of the reticuloendothelial tissue and the lymph system. Like all lymph glands, the solitary follicle and the Peyer's patches of the small and large intestines have a high silicon content. The greatest store of silicon found in the human body is in the glands, where silicon is apparently needed for developing their specific effects of activating phagocyte tissue elements."

Even before Ruge, Auer, Chief Physician for Inner Medicine in Frankfurt, Germany, stated that he had successfully treated typhoid conditions with silica in the 1930s. The preparation used was cited by Saller as "Siliquid." During treatments, neuralgia, neuritis, and migraines disappeared.

Baumeister recommended silica to relieve duodenal ulcer complaints in 21 days and gastritis after four days. Furuncles, whitlow, and burns healed. Wet eczema[20] and ulcera cruris, also leucorrhea and mastitis healed. Researcher H. Mahr in 1949 could favorably influence a young man's cervical gland tuberculosis.

K. H. Neuhoff successfully provided complete pain relief in eight to fourteen days with silica gel for patients with many forms of stomach illness. Saller, who ascribes silica's healing effect to the dependence on stimulation of appropriate connective tissue reactions, confirms this. The most difficult types of hemorrhoids also healed with silica gel.

Chronic or acute gastritis sufferers with repeated mucous membrane inflammations experience quick relief from accompanying troubles with oral doses of silica gel as a hot solution, pure or diluted. This complicated condition of chronic or acute gastritis often leads to distressing meteorism (bloating flatulence) that oppresses the heart through a high level of the midriff.

This may be surprising, but heart attacks can develop from such aggravated forms of meteorism. With silica gel therapy, constipation is present at the outset. This leads to increased stool pressure, but continued difficulty in eliminating the stool. Following rectal massage, a sheep-feces-like stool evacuates accompanied by cramped pressure. Stool pressure remains without greater amounts of stool being expelled. However, repeated oral doses of silica gel slowly lead to normalization. Dörre in his 1950 silica research could similarly improve gastritis with accompanying duodenal ulcer and ulcera ventriculi by prescribing silica gel treatment.

Facilitated Females
Women have some delicate problems in which silica gel can be of help. Supplementation has proven effective with discharge, abscesses and ulcers in the genital area and the cervix. It was found effective also in cases of mastitis, an inflammation of the mammary glands and the breasts. This is good news especially for breast feeding mothers. Talking of breasts brings up an interesting topic that I wish to clarify because of a close name association.

The Silly Silicone Scare and Silicosis
There is a distinct difference between silicon in the form of a watery silica gel and the highly controversial silicone breast implants that have become the focus of public attention. Silicone is not naturally found in body tissues. It is put there by doctors! Silicon is very different from silicone (with an "e" at the end) despite the close resemblance in name. The difference shows quite clearly when using chemical terms; unlike Si (silicon) in naturally occurring

compound forms like SiO_2 (silica) or H_4SiO_4, the silicic acid of silica gel, R_2SiO (silicone) is an industrial polymer where R is a hydrocarbon. Such hydrocarbons are suspected of being carcinogenic. A better and natural way for breast enhancement is simple supplementation with silica gel. This could help to reconstruct damaged tissue and thereby improve the breasts.

There also once was a public scare involving the element of silicon in dust particles breathed in primarily by miners. The resultant disorder was called silicosis. It has as little to do with the nutrient silica as the artificial silicone compound.

Conquering Cancer with Silica Gel
Cancer occurs mainly in middle and older ages, when the human body contains less silica. The activation of the body's defense stimulated by silica gel supplementation has a positive effect on cancer, although silica gel cannot be seen as a cancer-specific drug. It can be excellent as an underpinning supplementary therapy to cancer treatment. It can also be useful in cancer prevention therapy.

The Dunaris well in Daun, a small town in Germany, is again noteworthy in this context. The Daun county has the lowest cancer rate in western Europe. The water from the spring contains an abundance 80 mg per litre of silica! Sure enough, in 1932 researcher F. Goldstein incidently found that the county of Daun in the Eiffel region of Germany showed the lowest occurrence and mortality statistics for cancer.

Silica especially influences the degenerated white blood cells of cancer patients. It begins the regeneration of normal protein. With other biological cancer remedies, silica plays an important role in cancer therapy and in stopping the growth of malignant tumors. Even with the uncertainty of how silica proves its effectiveness, therapists, as will be seen, should make silica gel part of their treatment plan to help support the healing process.

Before 1936 little was known of the relationship between silica and cancer. In 1936, however, R. Willheim and K. Stern reported that the silica content of the pancreas increases in those afflicted with tumors and that elimination of silica through urination diminishes. Why would this be so? Does that mean silica supplementation is bad for cancer patients? However, researcher P. G. Seeger found that silicosis of the lungs that favors cancer formation is not "a specific carcinogenic effect attributable to silicon."

Researcher Kober traced cancer to a structural coarsening, reduction of boundary surfaces, and from that inferred the resultant inflammation. He agrees with the correlation between Domagk's view of cancer formation and that of diminishing atrophic tissue (i.e. with gum recession) and the resultant diminishing of the colloidal marginal surface.

In 1937-38 P. G. Seeger established in comparative vital color investigations of normal cells and ascites-carcinoma cells that, when cells become cancerous, a spongy loosening; i.e., swelling of mitochondria and of the cells occurs. The cancer problem a marginal cell surface problem.

Silica retrogressively influences the structural disintegration caused by carcinogens. It restores cell protein through prompting synthesis of normal protein bodies. Above all, it increases the number of defensive cells. The growth rate of cancer cells is inversely proportional to the number of defensive cells, as shown by Seeger and Schacht in 1957-58. Many others report successful treatment of carcinomas and sarcomas with silica. The correlation to deswelling of cell protein demonstrates silica, in its reversible influence on protein denaturing, to be an adjuvant as a prophylactic or in the therapy of malignant diseases.[21]

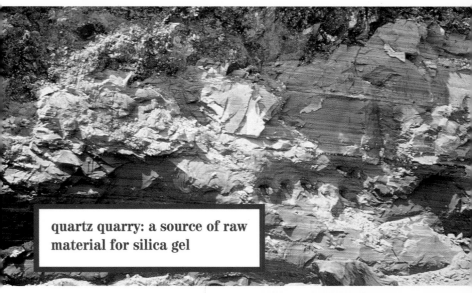

quartz quarry: a source of raw material for silica gel

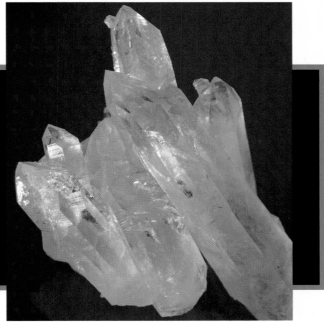

quartz is pure silica (silicon dioxide) in a crystal structure

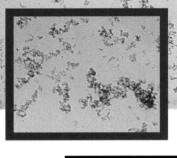

silica gel as seen through an electron microscope - the silica is highly dispersed and available to the body

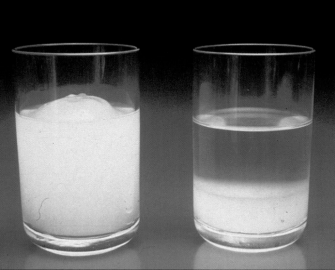

freezing temperatures destroy silica gel's structure: water and silica separate (right glass)

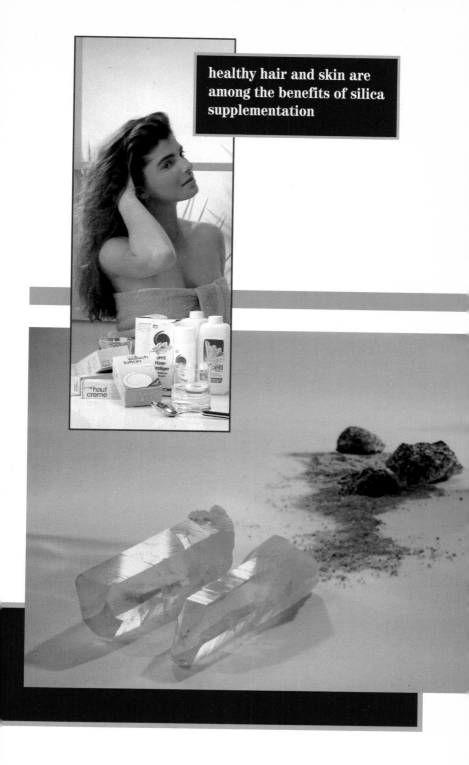

healthy hair and skin are among the benefits of silica supplementation

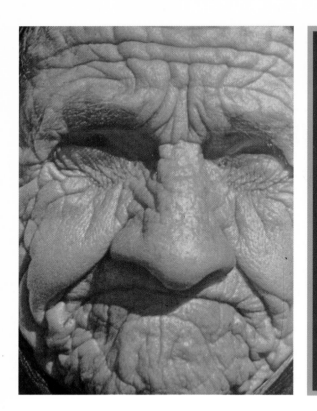

wrinkled skin occurs when connective tissue loses its ability to bind water

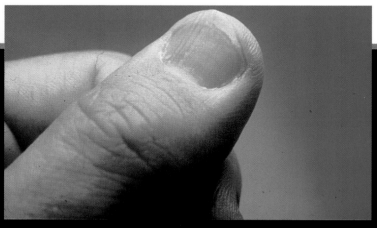

cracked, brittle nails suggest silica supplementation is needed

The effect of silica on cancer can thus be explained very easily. Silica has the characteristic of regenerating damaged and denatured protein through structural reintegration. Silica can inaugurate the synthesis of new albumin bodies. Silica's ability to activate mesenchymal connective tissue and lymph tissue and to increase the formation of lymphocytes and phagocytes is therefore of great importance in cancer therapy.

In view of this it is not surprising that silica was found by researcher Kober to be a chemotherapeutic. This means that silica is not a specific medicine against a certain disease that acts alone. Instead, with cancer it restores to the body an optimal colloid physical condition of tissue that guarantees the normal biological unfolding of the metabolic processes in cells.

This was confirmed through chemical analysis research in 1953 by H. Geiger. He became convinced that the colloidal effect, assuring the smooth flow of metabolic cell processes, was traceable to silica content. Geiger credited the silica-rich Dunaris water with great significance in the basic therapy of cancer. Researchers Lériche and Boncour also emphasize: "According to our experience, silica is one great basic medicine for the fight against cancer. It is important for mutations processes. It is indispensable for those ill with cancer as it is ever lacking in the organism's old age."

In this connection I find it tremendously interesting that silicon, that is present and required in the osteoblast cell which plays a decisive role in bone formation, was found in highest concentration in the mitochondria[22] of the osteoblast cell. The mitochondria, of course, is the cell's factory, so to speak.

Vascular Infirmity in Old Age

The most prevalent aging disorder is called arteriosclerosis (atherosclerosis is a form of arteriosclerosis) and is at the beginning of many vascular disorders. With silica gel supplementation, good circulation can be returned to aging circulatory systems. Dizziness, headache, buzzing in the ears and sleeping disorders, all consequences of arteriosclerotic damage, eventually disappear.

With silica, high blood pressure normalizes since the vascular walls become elastic and can again better adjust to their requirements. Atherosclerotic arteries contain 14 times less silica than healthy arteries. This was the finding of French researchers after studying 72 adults aged 61 and over. Silica is an effective and easy to tolerate biological remedy that not only suppresses symptoms but also improves the causes of atherosclerosis and arteriosclerosis and its consequences. Silica promotes artery impermeability to harmful lipids, preventing their deposits.

Silica's influence on vascular disease comes from its effect on the elastic connective tissue of vascular inner walls. A deswelling of vascular walls, especially the intima, with cholesterol storage and calcification, regeneration *ad integrum* can be achieved with silica.[23] Similarly, blood pressure decreases with hypertonia that comes from the same condition.

O. Scholl and K. Letters in 1959 examined the geriatric effect of silica. They were concerned with the 1958 findings of M. Bürger that bradytrophic tissue experiences a thickening process in advanced age. They confirmed the findings of colloid researcher M. H. Fischer that the precondition for all life processes occurring in plasma is the optimal water-combining and swelling of protein, corresponding to a 0.9 percent amount of NaCl.

They found that the primary process of aging rests upon dehydration. The resultant deswelling of protein is connected with alteration of osmosis and diffusion processes. This leads to flocculation and coagulation phenomena, i.e. denaturing of protein. The intima and media thicken with increased age with storage of intermediate substances, such as cholesterol and calcium stored in large plaques and cause a narrowing and hardening of the elastic vascular canals.

Gohr and Scholl in 1949 could halt and reverse these processes with one percent soluble silica and found that blood content increased from 0.7-1.1 percent after several weeks of treatment to 130 to 400 percent, while only 5.2 to 13.8 percent of the SiO_2 added was again in the urine. In experiments with artificially arteriosclerotic rats Scholl and Letters could, through feeding of sclerosol (colloidal silica gel), smooth through swelling and restore pink colour to shrivelled, brown colored kidney cells, i.e., normalize the cells.

In human studies, H. Gohr obtained a substantial improvement, disappearance of dizziness, ringing in the ears, sense of head pressure, and sleeplessness with 30 ml sclerosol daily after two months with 15 arteriosclerosis sufferers. Because of its regenerative effect, the use of silica for blood circulation disturbances works well. K. Kohler was successful in lowering fixed blood pressure in three patients from 240 to 160 mm with a combination of sclerosol and rauwolfia. Further human studies, including studies on comparative absorption rates and combining power (bioavailability) of colloidal silica gel are being planned by labs in Germany and the USA.

Aiding AIDS
How knowledgeable self-help and a sense of responsibility can safeguard personal health became vividly clear to me at the AIDS research program at Vancouver's St. Paul's Hospital, in which I assisted for some time. What emerged

most clearly for me from my contact with AIDS victims was that most of them had played fast and loose with their health, ignoring even simple safety precautions through years of reckless living. Stricken with disease, they suddenly saw that it takes a good guide to help the uninformed get out of the curative quagmires.

Yes, there is hope for HIV positive people. Silica influences the functioning of the entire immune system. It concentrates in the lymph nodes. There it exerts a positive influence on the functions of the lymphatic system. Its effects tremendously increase the production of phagocytes, the policing proteins. These specific enzymes kill germs and other foreign intruders.

People with inherent inferiority of the lymphatic system, a condition called lymphatic diatheses, can feel the uplifting effect of silica supplementation immediately. These people easily exhibit abnormal susceptibility to infectious disease. They suffer from chronically swollen lymph nodes, nervous disorders and fatigue. These symptoms are of special significance also in AIDS.

AIDS has been blamed exclusively on the HIV virus. However, a group of serious scientists, including the man who discovered the AIDS virus, now claim that the outbreak of AIDS can be prevented even in HIV positive people. The answer, they say, lies in strengthening the immune system. This is exactly what silica does.

Allowing even partial truth for the opinions of AIDS specialists, we can consider silica's immune system support activity as outstandingly beneficial in at least suppressing the outbreak of the active AIDS disease. To this extent it should recommend itself especially to people who are HIV positive and in whom the AIDS disease is not manifested.

I should imagine that, as often occurs in disease treatment, at the preventive stage silica gel promises the best therapeutic results. Nonetheless, silica supplementation seems to recommend itself to actual AIDS sufferers at least as an alternative and supplementary therapy.

It would require in-depth research (something I hope will happen) to figure out if silica can become central to HIV positive prevention or AIDS supplementary therapy. Silica offers hope for AIDS, but there is one specific degenerative disease in which silica has already proven itself to be of central importance. It is the subject of the next chapter.

Chapter Six

"The topic (La Silice et les Silicates) of my lectures to you has so far not received the attention it deserves."

Rudolf Wegscheider, Ph.D.
University of Vienna, 1919

Treating and Preventing Bone Thinning

Fractured Lives

Silicon plays an important role in protecting bones by aiding in the organic phase of bone mineralization, a process obviously gone awry in osteoporosis sufferers. The human frame is ably supported by many bones that comprise the skeleton structure so well-known to us from children's horror stories. Unlike the fictional figures in stories that become "living" skeletons, in osteoporosis, it is indeed the skeleton that is rapidly vanishing. This condition, if allowed to proceed unchecked, can cause bones to break suddenly without undue stress. It can quickly confine a person to a wheelchair.

Happily, bone thinning or osteoporosis can be prevented. The management of primary menopausal and senile osteoporosis lies in prevention. It is vital to work on prevention because today 15 million Americans are affected by osteoporosis. To find out if you have a potential problem with osteoporosis, ask your doctor to perform a bone density study. This is a non-invasive test (in Canada covered by Medicare). It is similar to an x-ray but far more specific in finding bone thinning. Without such a test you have no way of knowing where you stand and how far to go with diet and lifestyle changes. Once there is significant bone loss, it is difficult to reverse these debilitating forms of osteoporosis that make up 80 percent of cases, though silica administration offers some relief.*

Reduction in bone density is the result of the rate of bone resorption being greater than that of bone formation. Effects of aging, imbalance in hormonal secretions, long term calcium deficiency, lack of physical activity, acid ash diet and high phosphate diet are well-known factors. Newer findings point to the lack of other nutrients like magnesium, phosphorus, vitamin C, boron, and last but not least, silicon, which exerts a balancing effect on bone calcium.

According to Nancy Appleton, Ph.D.,[24] other detrimental factors include the consumption of sugar, excessive stress, caffeine, tobacco and alcohol, a high protein diet and drugs such as aspirin, antibiotics, and antacids. Some of these can also be seen as detrimental lifestyle factors. Since the cause is multifarious, treatment is symptomatic. The outlook for long-term therapy for post-menopausal osteoporosis is good. What should long-term therapy consist of? Let us explore the various forms of orthodox and alternative treatments available to combat osteoporosis.

Unwanted Side Effects of Drugs
Many women take oestrogen pills to prevent osteoporosis. However, estrogen and similar dangerous drugs cannot qualify for prevention and self-treatment. Other current hormonal research focuses on progesterone, which may slow bone loss by boosting bone density in women before menopause. Another hormonal treatment involves calci-

---

* Secondary osteoporosis, making up 20 percent, has different causes, relates to other disorders and requires special medical attention. It is not addressed here.

tonin. This hormone is a regulator of the level of calcium present in the blood at any one time. This regulatory hormone is now synthesized. Canada prohibits the treatment of primary osteoporosis with synthetic calcitonin. The USA, Italy, Spain and Japan allow prescription use.

The drug must be injected, much like insulin. Calcitonin combats bone thinning much as oestrogen does. It is based on the concept that bone rebuilds if the two processes – reabsorbing old bone and forming new bone – are balanced. Both oestrogen and calcitonin slow down bone resorption. Calcitonin apparently also eases bone pain. Both drugs cause unwanted side effects.

A study completed in August 1992 at the University of Utah found that the drinking of fluoridated water leads to greater incidence of fractures among older people. Though not claiming certainty because of conflicting studies, this is obviously one more good reminder to all people, regardless of their current age, to avoid drinking fluoridated water whenever possible in order to avert a later backlash for their health.

Lifestyle and Exercise Factors
Zoltan P. Rona, M.D., M.Sc., points out that "increased risk factors for the development of osteoporosis include cigarette smoking, excessive alcohol and caffeine intake, having a fair complexion, having had the ovaries removed or other causes of early menopause, a positive family history of osteoporosis, never having been pregnant, drugs such as cortisone, diuretics (water pills), anti-seizure medications and anticoagulants (blood thinners), digestive disorders and overactive endocrine glands (especially hyperthyroidism). He agrees that daily exercise throughout the active years is perhaps the best osteoporosis prevention.

On the other hand, excessive exercise of female athletes who push too hard to be slim and excel in their sport, may result in the reduction of female hormone production. This risk, often accompanied by amenorrhea (lack of periods), is greatest in high-pressured gymnastics. Coaches, parents and female athletes should understand the real risk of causing premature bone thinning through such over-rigorous exercise. The message is clear: compete, but don't compete to the detriment of your health.

The Calcium Factor

Silicon researcher Günther Lindemann epitomized the interdependent connection between calcium and silica when he said that "we are secured between the polar powers of silica and calcium. While our skin is woven into the universality of silica, through our skeleton we are connected to the calcium process of earthly-mineral solidity."

A 1992 double-blind study by Dr. C. Conrad Johnston Jr. and colleagues using identical twins at Indiana University showed that young children grow denser bones if they double their calcium intake. However, even these experts, despite their findings, question whether children should consume more calcium. Researchers found that kids who get about 1,600 mg of calcium a day – equivalent to 1.3 quarts of milk – had measurably denser bones than those who consumed just over 800 mg, just over the recommended dosage. If the extra bone density persists through life, it could protect against bone thinning. However, only pre-pubescent youngsters appeared to benefit from the extra calcium.

In an editorial the *New England Journal of Medicine* cautions against loading children up with extra calcium until more is known about extra calcium's long term effects. No one knows how long the extra bone density may last as people grow older. Further research is indicated before giving normal children and adolescents large doses of calcium. This is emphasized by the fact that those who arrived at puberty during the three year study or were already into adolescence when it started, showed no measurable difference.

As for adults, in the first volume, *Silica – The Forgotten Nutrient,* I have challenged the unquestioned use of calcium supplementation by adults and have shown its interdependence with silica. Calcium is still most closely linked with osteoporosis management. Yet no research has definitely shown that supplemental calcium can increase bone tissue mass or prevent osteoporotic fractures or collapse. The normal serum calcium level is 80.5 – 10.3 mg/l, or 4.2 – 5.1 mEq/L (2.1-2.6 mmol/L). Calcium supplementation is a rule in the management of osteoporosis, but calcium is another mineral that is difficult to absorb. The chief regulator of intestinal calcium intake is vitamin D that also plays a role in bone formation.* Studies at UCLA showed far less osteoblasts in the skull bone matrix of baby chicks fed a vitamin D deficient test diet.

Unfortunately, the human body's exact daily requirement of calcium is unknown and given as between 300 and 1,500 mg . The Recommended Daily Allowance (RDA) is 800 mg daily for adults. It is 1,200 for adolescents and pregnant and lactating mothers. After age 60, less calcium is absorbed from the diet by both sexes, making calcium supplementation advisable.

The Silicon Factor

Silica, it has been shown, is a major player in keeping bones solid although it does not appear to be so at first sight. That is because bones consist mainly of calcium, magnesium and

---

* Lack of vitamin D in children leads to bone deformities, a deficiency disease called rickets.

phosphate. But they also contain silica, which is important for the deposition of mineral salts, especially calcium.

Silicon in silica acts similarly to vitamin D in the hastening of bone formation. This is so no matter which bones are formed. Silicon is involved in the organic stage of bone formation, even of skull bones, which are formed differently from other bones in which cartilage is turned into bone. Silicon is, according to Professor Carlisle, uniquely localized in the osteogenic layer of bone tissue. There the presence of silicon helps to continuously produce new bone tissue in the bone matrix.

Dr. Carlisle, using "in vivo" studies of chicks and rats, also confirmed that silica nutrients are essential for strong bones, cartilage and the combs of chicks. The studies with baby chicks on silicon-poor diets showed that silicon deficiency leads to less calcified bones. I find it revealing of silicon's role that mucopolysaccharides, which enable living tissue to hold water, are a common factor in the tissue in chick combs, collagen and bones.

In a 1986 x-ray microanalysis, Dr. Carlisle reported active growth in young bone and isolated osteoblasts, showing silicon to be a major ion of osteogenic cells. The amounts of silicon found in osteoblast cells are in the same range as that of calcium, phosphorus, and magnesium. Carlisle found silicon to be especially high in the metabolically active state of the osteoblast. This is clear evidence that silicon is required for connective and bone tissue matrix formation.

Bones containing high silicon levels also contained correspondingly high calcium levels.* Silicon supplementation hastened the rate of bone mineralizing. As shown in "in vivo" tests, silicon supplementation did so especially in test

---

* The UCLA studies also showed that when silicon and calcium were lower in certain other cells, phosphorus was higher.

animals kept on a low calcium diet. The UCLA "in vivo" findings are corroborated by later "in vitro" findings in which skull and other bones were grown in petri dishes. Those without silicon in the growth medium grew hardly any collagen, again showing the tremendous importance of silicon in collagen (and therefore in bone formation).

It is known that in human females with post-menopausal calcium loss, silica depletes. The presence of silica effects healing of bone fractures and callus formation. It functions as a remineralizing agent and prepares for recalcification. In corroboration of Carlisle's findings, researchers Charnot and Rabat found a complete silica deficiency in bones with bone softening in a disease endemic to North Africa. Canadian author Dr. Zoltan Rona sees nothing incompatible between calcium citrate and silica. He points out that silica is concentrated in the body in sites of active calcification in the bones, as previously also determined by researchers Passwater and Cranton.

Perhaps the long-term detrimental effect of PTH (parathyroid hormone) combined with inhibited or poor calcium absorption is a major contributing factor of osteoporosis. If so, could supplementation with silica gel achieve better calcium absorption and thereby cancel the long-term resorption of precious bone mass? Clearly, more research is needed on how to overcome the detriments of PTH effects.

Yet even now it seems a logical conclusion that given calcitonin's short-term regulation, the long-term PTH factor may be the key to osteoporosis. Aside from its villainy role in osteoporosis, PTH is a necessary and natural hormonal function of the body with the vital task of maintaining serum calcium equilibrium. It therefore cannot be inhibited or prevented from the detrimental effects it has on bones. It follows that supplementation with silica seems the only wise choice to prevent osteoporosis and brittle bones, commonly experienced in older people.

Bone thinning develops from inadequate silica, vitamin D, vitamin C, calcium, magnesium, manganese, copper and zinc according to Robert A. Anderson, M.D.[25] He found that musculoskeletal injuries during athletic training occur in athletes who have significantly lower levels (four ppm) of silicon as determined by hair analysis. This contrasts with subjects who train without injury and show normal levels of silicon in their hair, i.e., over 20 ppm.

According to Dr. Daniel B. Mowrey, "in experimental settings involving the effect of silicon on bone growth, most of the increase in growth appeared to be due to a rise in collagen content. Similar results have been demonstrated in the growth of cartilage." By the way, you would not want to loose your cartilage tissue. It is a special tissue that can hold large amounts of water due to the presence of mucopolysaccharides* and protein network that acts like a sponge. Cartilage is an excellent example of a tissue in which silicon has a dual role of structure and metabolism. The body makes cartilage primarily to act as a cushion between joints of the bones.

A good example of a cartilage cushion preventing the rubbing together of harder bone plates is the knee joint. My mother-in-law, who lives in Germany, has much trouble with her knees. She suffers from osteoarthritis, a chronic condition and degenerative disease that often leads to the loss of cartilage and inhibits joint movement. Her knees often hurt because of lost cartilage. She has new hope since her last visit with us for Christmas 1991 because she is now supple-

---

* The prefix "muco" very aptly indicates their watery nature. However, biochemistry now prefers to call them glucominoglycanes.

menting her diet with silica. Silicon from silica is another important constituent of the mucopolysaccharides, enabling them to hold water.

Cartilage and collagen are both intimately associated with bone formation. However, Dr. Mowrey[26] suggests that if bone, cartilage and collagen are involved in an injury, the body's repair functions give bone repair precedence over the other functions. That is another way of saying that there is bone repair impairment in the absence of silica. This constitutes the ultimately clear proof that silica intake is bone-essential!

Chapter Seven

"For nothing is secret, that shall not be made manifest; neither any thing hid, that shall not be known and come abroad."

King James Bible, Luke 8:17

Continuous Colloidal Care Wakes a Tired Metabolism

Gel Works

The single molecules of silica form a firming structure that supports and helps tissue where tissue metabolism and rejuvenation take place. The effectiveness of silica gel for the immune system comes from the activation of phagocytes – a kind of "health police" – in our blood and lymphatic circulation. Bacteria and germs are killed to help our system fight off illness.

Silica gel's organic absorption rate has been intensively and conclusively tested. Of particular fascination is a 1989 resorption study of the Medical Clinic of the University of Freiburg, done by Dr. J. Thiele and Dr. E. Bisse under the direction of Prof. Dr. N. Katz. The study employed laboratory rats. The method allowed for the quantitative tracing of organic silica of up to 90 percent (something that is extremely difficult to achieve) in the test animals.

Test animals were given supplemental colloidal silica gel of 0.07 and 0.17 ml (0.63 percent and 1.54 percent of total silica supply) in addition to their regular Eggermanns optimal rat diet (containing 4.4 mg silica per gram). This means an average silica supply of 100 mg for a rat with a body weight of 300 g.

Rats given supplemental colloidal silica gel showed a tendency to eat less than the control group. Their blood silica levels were nevertheless by 29.5 percent>17 percent or significantly *higher* than the controls. Even more astounding, the researchers found that the absorption rate of silica in feed versus supplemented silica gel was different. Colloidal mineral silica gel appeared to enter the bloodstream quicker, pointing to a greater intestinal absorption rate.

These amazingly positive metabolic assimilation values for colloidal silica gel conclusively prove its bioavailability. The results were further corroborated by analysis of silica content of certain body organs. Whole blood showed an increase of 13 ug/ml to 23 ug/ml following administration of consecutive doses of 0.07 ml/day and 0.17 ml/day over three days.

It is also interesting that the silica concentration in blood serum was markedly lower than in whole blood. This indicates that a quicker diffusion of silica happens through the erythrocytic membrane. In other organs silica was found primarily in the lungs, liver and spleen. It is important to note that organs in these organ analyses showed remarkable differences between the test rats and the controls whereas no such dissimilarities were found in blood serum and the heart.

Beautifying Hair, Skin and Nails from Within and Without
The most fault-finding and analytical member of our family is my sister-in-law Titia. She came to visit us from Vienna, Austria. We had not seen her in years and there was much joy being reunited. Particularly so as I was celebrating my 50th birthday. On the second day following her arrival we were all comfortably seated in the sunshine on the back

porch—Titia suddenly looked quizzically at me, then asked bemused, "Tell me, Klaus, do you dye your hair?" "No," I replied perplexed. "Well," Titia continued, "that's very astounding. You don't have any grey hair!" "There are a few," I ventured modestly, "they are just hidden." "No, give me the truth," she chuckled. "The truth?" I echoed slowly. Then I said, "Truth is: I am supplementing with silica. You are looking at the results of long-term preventive silica therapy. And I add weekly external silica gel packs for increased efficiency."

Hair, skin and nails are the most visible parts of our body. We want them to be beautiful because they play such an important role in how we view our health image. Their appearance affects how we feel, how we look at ourselves and how we relate to others in a social context. They also are truly important to our well-being. If asked to point out the largest organ of the body, would you say the liver? You would be dead wrong. The correct answer would be the skin —the body's largest organ. Skin, hair and nails are the living cover that often shows on the outside how well off we are within. The presence of silica in our body can maintain the lustre in our hair, the strength in our nails, the tone of our skin.

When I revealed that I had not had a cold in years, Titia asked me to get her a long-term supply of silica gel and also of vegetal silica to take back to Vienna because, she said "you never know if I can get these silica products in Austria. Besides for my hair, skin and nails, I can also use strengthening of my immune system. I get far too many colds." How simple it can be to turn a critical family member into a health-conscious and prevention-caring individual.

Truly, silica gel can care for the skin in a unique way like no other skin care. It is a general tonic that increases the strength and elasticity against all kinds of negative influences. Unlike most skin care products, silica can be used internally and externally. It has a double action on damaged skin by restoring skin vitality from within to without and from without to within.

Skin is absorptive as shown by Dr. Horrobin and prosta-glandins research that found Efamol good for baby skin as it penetrates into the body and is especially essential for babies who do not receive mother's milk. In such babies, it can act as a substitute for mother's milk. In the skin, large sugars similar to the ones found in cartilage (mucopolysac-charides) combine with protein and form a network that enables the skin to hold water. The water-binding ability is helped by the presence of silicon and hiuronic acid (often contained in cosmetics). Without this ability to hold water, your skin would quickly become wrinkly. This points to a silica loss in aged skin and the restorative value of silicon supplementation for skin.

Externally, silica is effective for itching, rashes, abscesses, boils, acne, calluses, warts, eczema, corns, benign skin sores, insect bites and bed sores. Skin injuries, burns and frostbite heal quicker and without complications. Ulcers (including varicose ulcers) can be positively influenced by silica. Already many years ago, the Austrian cancer specialist and healer Rudolf Breuss advocated ingestion and bathing in silica-rich alpine horsetail for the effective treatment of varicose ulcers. He ascribed the healing effect to its high content of silicic acid.

Older research confirms that silica is present in many dif-ferent epithelial structures.[27] In 1901, researcher Hugo Schulz arrived at the view that there could be no connective tissue without silica. Medicine testing by that same researcher shows that silica obtains the best therapeutic results with all forms of acne. It also clears up insect bites, solid infiltrating furuncles, pustular rashes, sweat gland abscesses, necrotic processes such as decubitus, hair loss, paronychia (nail-bed infection) and finger nail breakage. J. Mezger finds silica to be the best means for treatment of scar keloid, foot callouses, warts, lipomas, ganglia, fibromas, corns, furuncles and burns.

According to C. P. Unna, silica raises the skin's resistance ability and promotes formation of protective, lining body tissues, especially covering skin tissue, i.e., epithelialisation. In 1930, M. Kochmann and L. Maier showed that the skin elasticity of white mice can be improved by inserting silica solution by oral ingestion and subcutaneous injection combined. Studies undertaken in the former Soviet Union revealed a slowing of hair loss through silica therapy.

Using Silica Gel
An ideal silica supplement would be easy to take (swallow), easy to absorb (metabolize), convenient to store (keep) and easy to remember to take. Colloidal silica gel answers all these demands. Silica gel can be handily stored in the refrigerator in easy reach. Silica gel can be ingested undiluted with the help of a spoon or can be diluted in a glass of water. It has a pleasant, neutral taste.

Silica gel, taken like a juice or syrup, is extremely easy to ingest, especially for people who experience difficulties swallowing pills or capsules. One tablespoon of silica gel covers an area of three square meters. This large reactive area offers lots of opportunities for biological interaction inside the body's colloidal tissues.

Silica gel should be kept in a cool place. A bottle of silica gel, once it is opened, should be refrigerated (but not below 40°F or 4°C). Silica gel is most conveniently located in your fridge. Every time you open the fridge and see it, you will

93

be reminded not to forget your daily silica supplement. I find that it works like a charm.

Tonic Uses

As a tonic, one tablespoon of the gel is ingested three times daily over a period of one to two months. For this purpose the gel should be diluted in two ounces of mineral water. You can substitute herbal tea, your favorite fruit juice or other beverage. Tonic treatment is best taken in-between mealtimes.

It has been found that the therapeutic effect of nutrients often improves after discontinuing usage for some time. After a three month interval, treatment can be repeated. Pause and repetition both help to stabilize the effect. Of course, silica gel use can be extended for longer periods and the breaks can be varied depending on therapeutic aims. In case of doubt, ask your practitioner.

Prescriptions for Internal Uses

Weakness of the Connective Tissue

Ingest one tablespoon of silica gel diluted in tea or water as a daily supplement. It supports the connective tissue and helps prevent damage.

Stiff/Pulled Ligaments – Damaged Disks

Take one tablespoon silica gel diluted in tea or yogurt over a period of about three months.

Hair Loss

Take one to two tablespoons of silica gel diluted in mineral water over a period of three months.

Brittle Nails

Take one tablespoon of silica gel daily in tea or water over a longer period.

Flabby Skin

Take one to two tablespoons of silica gel diluted in mineral water over a period of three to four months for a sufficient supply of silica.

Aging and Aging Disorders

Ingest one tablespoon silica gel diluted in tea over several months.

Bone Structure

The elemental substance silica acts as a "tractor" function for the calcium deposition in bones. Therefore, during growth periods after bone fractures, silica helps support the body and speed the healing process. Take one tablespoon silica gel diluted in mineral water per day during the recovery period.

Strengthening the Body's Immune System

Silica promotes the formation of phagocytes and lymphocytes. These two cell varieties are important to our immune systems and help us become less susceptible to infections and toxins. Take one tablespoon silica gel diluted in mineral water. With a silica deficiency, it is recommended to use the preparation over a longer period. It is good to know that there are no drawbacks or side effects known for long-term use of colloidal mineral silica gel.

Chronic or acute gastritis

With repeated mucous membrane inflammations experience quick relief from accompanying troubles with oral doses as a hot solution, pure or diluted. Repeated oral doses of silica gel slowly lead to normalization.

Gastrointestinal Tract

For problems of the gastrointestinal tract, take one tablespoon of silica gel after meals with five times as much liquid. Acute problems might disappear after the first usage; otherwise repeat every two to three hours. For chronic problems, use several weeks.

External Affairs

Colloidal silica gel has the ability to bind bacteria, germs, and wound secretions. The colloidal silica is absorbed very well by injured skin and stimulates the growth of new tissue. This dual activity of silica gel speeds up wound healing.

Connective tissue and with it vascular walls are strengthened through silica absorption through the tissue membranes.

When using silica gel externally, keep in mind the physical law that heat disperses while cold congeals or inhibits reabsorption of an effusion. So, repeated hot bandaging with diluted silica gel is very successful with sprains, dislocations, pulled muscles with or without bleeding, joint inflammations, infiltrates under the skin, and insect bites.

It follows that silica gel has a positive effect on chronic purulence. Applying warm bandaging to purulent processes such as furunculosis, nail bed inflammations, phlegmon, abscesses, and mastitis has a similar healing effect. Skin rashes, eczema, whether itching, moist, dry, inflamed or pus-producing, are all healed more quickly by hot wrapping.

Wraps should be applied twice a day, each time for half an hour. Hot compresses should be renewed every three to four minutes and then be covered with a wool cloth or thick cotton towel. Repeat moist and warm wrapping often, clean and dry the wounds to promote the healing process. In case of danger of a pus eruption toward the inside, it is suggested to consult your physician first to decide whether the focus must be opened prior to application of silica gel.

Hemorrhoidal complaints can be alleviated by external application of a cotton ball saturated with undiluted silica gel. Mucous membrane inflammation of the mouth and pharynx, such as stomatitis, angina, and laryngitis respond well to gargling or rinsing with diluted silica gel. This should be accompanied by oral doses. For external treatment of skin problems silica gel can be dabbed on undiluted, several times daily. Another way of treating appropriate skin areas would be to dilute one tablespoon of silica gel with four tablespoons of water and applied as a compress that can be remoistened two to three times from the outside before removal. This can be done up to four times daily.

Quick Healing from One to Nine

The following unique application and treatment observations are from the interesting patient records of Dr. Baumeister, M.D., a practicing physician of Herne, Westphalia, in Germany. I found his nine points or observations useful in formulating particular or additional silica supplementation. They also confirm the use of silica in the medical practice:

1. *Internal Medicine*

   Silica has experienced a changeable fate in medicine. It has undergone constant experiments since the time of Paracelsus. For enteric colitis, summer cholera, allergic irritant conditions of the intestinal tract, typhoid, gastritis, including ulcus-ventriculi-complex, take internally two to three times per day one teaspoon in some water, eventually higher doses, also as an enema one tablespoon in 1/2 liter of water. For long term use twice a day one teaspoon to one tablespoon. In cases of arteriosclerosis with hypertonia (aging disease), meteorism use three to five times a day one tablespoon pure.

2. *Surgery*

   With furuncles (moist compresses in dilutions of 1:3 to 1:10), abscesses, purulent infections under the skin (phlegmon), wound cleaning and healing, hemorrhoids.

3. *Dermatology*

   With dermatitis, wet eczema, ulcus cruris, pre-decubitus and decubitus, itching, burns of all degrees, insect bites, frostbite.

4. *Gynaecology and Obstetrics*

   With childbed mammary gland inflammation (puerperal mastitis), Bartholin's abscesses, white vaginal discharge (fluor albus), portio erosion (tampon application).

5. *Pediatrics*
   With soreness, chicken pox.
6. *Ear, Nose and Throat*
   With mucous membrane catarrh, hearing canal furuncles, paranasal sinus suppurations (rinse), otitis (drops).
7. *Ophthalmology*
   With connective tissue catarrh (dilute 1:10).
8. *Stomatology and Tooth, Mouth, and Maxillary Medicine*
   With stomatitis, pharynx catarrh, gingivitis, alveolar-pyor-rhoea, parodontitis (rinse, mouthwash), gangrene (paste filling).
9. *Urology*
   With cystitis (rinse) (dilute 1:3).

Baumeister's guidelines are worthy of attention. Without hesitation though, by far the quickest and most comprehensive way of obtaining a good working knowledge of silica gel for prevention and therapy is the topic of the next chapter.

Chapter Eight

"A textbook is not an energy carrier, but a catalyst."
Wilhelm Ostwald, Ph.D.
Colloidal Researcher (1853–1932)

The Healing Journey
of 73 in '72

Empirical Overview

Silica gel's uses are multi-faceted and more numerous than those of horsetail-derived silica. Silica gel was formulated to be applied also externally. The extensive empirical data I found on the benefits of silica gel could easily fill a third volume on silica. For this reason, much of the available research data could not be included. I have restricted myself to including only the most relevant study.

The given case histories have great significance as reference models for practitioners and as self-help pointers for lay people. The histories are firsthand reflections of silica's healing impact. Nothing can be more convincing. The "in vivo" case studies have an immediacy, an urgency, that is impossible to obtain from laboratory "in vitro" studies. This data bank can be used time and again.

In 1990, researcher E. Blaurock-Busch reported increased values of the silica content in the hair, nails and blood of 22 subjects tested with silica gel. In 1983 (as per R. Graf) 15 patients with stomach and intestinal disorders were treated with silica gel. The study shows excellent digestibility and tolerance to silica gel with good therapeutic results.

Also in a 1983 study, A. Gegeckas reported quick and reliable relief from silica gel for 17 patients with stomach and intestinal problems. E. Dörling, in 1979, reported of 12 patients treated over 12 weeks. They showed 70 percent nail improvements, 60 percent stomach complaints alleviation and 73 percent improved digestion. In 1978, 40 patients with various dermatological disorders were treated with silica gel, resulting in significant therapeutic successes as reported by F. Fegeler. In 1976, J. Messerich reported a study of 71 patients with intestinal-stomach problems that resulted in 62 percent excellent, 14.1 percent good and 15.5 percent satisfactory therapeutic effects.[29]

German Patients Study
Important medical trials on silica deficiency states were done between 1972 and 1990. A number of significant field studies were done in Germany (then West Germany) with the special compound silicea-Balsam.[*] This form of silica was selected because it contains silica (silicon dioxide SiO_2) (German: Kieselsäure[†]) in an extremely finely-dispersed, colloidal form from which (compound[‡]) form silicon (German: Silizium) can be optimally assimilated and used. One hundred ml of silicea-Balsam contains 2.8 g silicic acid-anhydride in precipitated form.

* This coined trade name describes a colloidal silica with emollient or balm-like qualities. Manufactured by: Anton Hübner GmbH, Postfach 49, D-7801 Ehrenkirchen 1, Germany. In Canada and the USA this has since been renamed "Body Essential Silica Gel," a registered trademark.

† The original German text employs a term that should be translated into silicic acid (SiO_2nH_2O or other variety of silicic acids such as orthosilicic acid or tetraoxosilicic acid). However, the original text also describes "Kieselsäure" as SiO_2, making the correct translation term: silica.

‡ The definition "compound" is being added by this translator as silicon atoms do not occur in free form (on earth).

Completion of the Field Study

Seventy-three patients participated in this field study, of which 39 (53.42 percent) were women and 34 (46.5 percent) men. The youngest participant was 24, the oldest 76 years of age, with an averaga age of 52.37 years. The treatment cycle lasted from 14 days to 4.25 months, averaging 1.97 months.

Colloidal mineral silica gel was applied according to the following findings:

14 patients	(19.1%)	arteriosclerosis and its successive stages
9 patients	(12.33%)	bronchial catarrh, bronchitis
14 patients	(19.1%)	cold, cough, pharyngeal catarrh, laryngeal catarrh
5 patients	(6.5%)	connective tissue weakness
3 patients	(4.11%)	lymphadenopathy, lymphatic diathesis
9 patients	(12.33%)	stomatitis (oral mucosa inflammation), gingivitis (gum inflammation), ulorrhoea (gum bleeding), ulatrophy (gum recession)
6 patients	(0.22%)	gastroenteritis, diarrhea, flatulence
13 patients	(17.0%)	skin, hair and nail disease/injury
73 patients	(100.0%)	in total

Within the framework of this present study silica gel was administered as follows:

Internal Daily dosage one to two times one tablespoon in water for arteriosclerosis, bronchial catarrh, bronchitis, cough, pharyngeal catarrh, lymphadenopathy, lymphatic diathesis, skin (dermatitis), hair (trichosis) and nail disease; in acute gastroenteritis every two hours until improvement one tablespoon pure, after that until recovery the preceding daily dose.

External Daily dosage one to three times applied in pure state; in dressings and compresses one to four times daily in ratio 1:3, applied diluted with water; for colds three to six times undiluted or snorted in 1:2 diluted with water; for gargling and mouth washes two to four times daily used 1:3 diluted with water; external treatment was used for colds, pharyngeal and/or laryngeal catarrh, stomatitis, gingivitis, ulatrophy, dermatosis (skin disease) and injuries.

No other medicines that could influence the test results were prescribed. None were used by the patients for self-help.

Test Results
Silica gel achieved excellent to satisfactory treatment results in 64 patients (87.67%). In seven patients (9.59%) the therapeutic results were average. Only in two cases (2.74%) was there no noticeable effect.

The total results can be decoded as follows:

13 patients	(17.0%)	excellent efficacy
28 patients	(38.36%)	good efficacy
23 patients	(31.51%)	satisfactory efficacy
7 patients	(9.59%)	ordinary efficacy
2 patients	(2.74%)	no significant efficacy
73 patients	(100.0%)	in total

Decoding according to the individual field of application yields the following detailed test results of this field study.

Efficacy	Arteriosclerosis		Bronchial Catarrh, Bronchitis		Gastroenteritis Disease		Skin/Hair/Nail	
excellent	2 cases	(14.29%)	1 case	(11.11%)	1 case	(16.67%)	2 cases	(15.3%)
good	4 cases	(2.57%)	3 cases	(33.33%)	3 cases	(50.00%)	5 cases	(3.46%)
satisfactory	5 cases	(35.71%)	4 cases	(44.44%)	1 case	(16.57%)	4 cases	(30.77%)
ordinary	2 cases	(14.29%)	1 case	(11.11%)	1 case	(16.67%)	2 cases	(15.3%)
insignificant	1 case	(7.14%)	0 cases	(0.0%)	0 cases	(0.0%)	0 cases	(0.0%)
Total	14 cases	(100.0%)	9 cases	(100.0%)	6 cases	(100.0%)	13 cases	(100%)

Efficacy	Colds, Coughs Pharynx, Larynx		Connective Tissue Weakness		Lymphatic Lymphadenopathy		Oral, Gum Disease	
excellent	3 cases	(21.43%)	1 case	(20%)	1 case	(33.33%)	2 cases	(22.22%)
good	5 cases	(35.71%)	3 cases	(60%)	1 case	(33.33%)	4 cases	(44.44%)
satisfactory	5 cases	(35.71%)	1 case	(20%)	0 cases	(0%)	3 cases	(33.33%)
ordinary	1 case	(7.14%)	0 cases	(0.0%)	0 cases	(0.0%)	0 cases	(0.0%)
insignificant	0 cases	(0.0%)	0 cases	(0.0%)	1 case	(33.33%)	0 cases	(0.0%)
Total	14 cases	(100%)	5 cases	(100%)	3 cases	(100%)	9 cases	(100%)

These outstanding results convincingly confirm the above-average efficacy of silica gel within the areas of application tested by this field study. Especially highlighted in this study is the effect on mucous membrane infections of the upper respiratory air passages, of the mouth, and in gum disease.

All patients tolerated silica gel very well; undesired side effects or attending symptoms appeared in no cases, not even in long-term therapy. Following the summary, I will list the results and the treatment course of all individual cases.

Summary
The study covers a test with silica gel (silicea-Balsam), in which 73 patients participated. On the average, they were treated for 1.97 months based on the following diagnosis:

- arteriosclerosis and its consequences;
- bronchial catarrh, bronchitis, colds, coughs, laryngeal and pharyngeal catarrh;
- connective tissue weakness;
- lymphadenopathy, lymphatic diathesis;
- stomatitis;
- gum infections, gum bleeding, recession;
- gastrointestinal illness, flatulence, diarrhea
- skin, hair, nail disease, injuries.

Silica gel was applied internally or externally, pure or diluted with water, for dressings, poultices, mouth and nose rinses, and for gargling always by the method prescribed. Other medicines that could influence the test results were not prescribed and not used for self-help.

In a convincing 87.67 percent of cases the silica therapy proved very good to satisfactorily effective. In 9.59 percent, fair results were still achieved, and only in 2.74 percent of cases no appreciable improvement resulted.

Especially in mucous membrane infections of the upper respiratory tract, of the mouth and the gums, the test yielded better than average, very good, and good therapeutic results. Outstanding therapeutic results were also achieved in other indications. The tolerance level to silica gel was very good in all patients, even when the remedy was administered for months.

Individual Therapeutic Indications

The broad range of silica gel potency makes silica gel apparent as (with all reservations that can be advanced against this kind of "cure-all" designation) a kind of elixir that is at least suggested for basic therapy in many disease states. Simultaneously silica gel remains – on the premise of compliance of methodology of course – free of undesired side effects and concomitant phenomena even in long term applications. We can conclude that it is also well suited as a modern household remedy.

Connective Tissue Weakness

Connective tissue designates those support structures whose intracellular substance cannot be stressed through pressure. Connective tissue consists of collagen, elastin and mucopolysaccharide (also named glucominoglycane). Silica is present in all of these tissues. Connective tissue cells are branched and remain in connection with each other through fine flagellums. Besides these resting cells there are in most kinds of connective tissue (primarily in the reticulum) wandering cells that variously serve body defence.

The intracellular substance of the connective tissue outweighs the regular cell substance. Only in fatty tissue, whose cells are puffed up by fat deposits, the cell mass outweighs the connective tissue. The intracellular substance includes the hydrous matrix, that contains silica in particular abundance also, and the fibers cradled therein are also silica-rich.

105

In principle one differentiates three kinds of fibers:

- collagen (glutinous), with stress or stretch qualities, that make up the building protein and are present in all connective and support tissue.
- grid fibers, the gossamer fibers of connective tissue, that at the periphery between connective tissue and the most superficial skin and mucous membrane layers make up two-dimensional, in the reticular connective tissue three-dimensional, lattice works.
- elastic fibers, that can branch and form everywhere where elasticity of the tissue is required, for instance in the arterial walls and the lungs.

The following tissue structures belong to connective tissues:

- loose connective tissue, that makes possible the sliding of organs against each other.
- fatty tissue, that serves as a storage organ, partially also as support tissue (hand and foot covering).
- taut-fibrous, stretchable connective tissue, for instance the tendons.
- reticular connective tissue that predominates in the spleen and the lymph system. It contains three-dimensionally arranged lattice fibers with wandering cells in the reticulate lace work of the grid and is primarily responsible for body defense.
- mesenchyme tissue, an embryonic (immature) fluid-filled spongy tissue, from which all cells of the connective tissue originate. It forms a kind of reservoir for cells.

As connective tissue permeates the entire body and participates in numerous functions, dysfunction also negatively affects the entire organism. Such a connective tissue weakness is often connected to the individual's genetic code, but is connected foremost to silica deficiency. Usually the victims are slender-built archetypes of infirm body posture and puffed up skin. Often lymphadenopathy is simultaneously present.

Their connective tissue is weakly developed, in particular tendons, articular capsules and muscle sarcolemma. For that reason, sprains, dislocations, pulling, overstretching and intestinal hernias (abdominal wall too delicate) often develop. The stomach can be uncinate and sunken into the remaining intestines, so that they reach deep into the pelvis, which also leads to significant dysfunction. The narrow thoracic cage constricts the lungs, rendering them badly oxygenated with a tendency to functional disturbances. Most often, too, the veins emerge clearly. Many stricken suffer from varicose veins or hemorrhoids. Lastly, the connective tissue weakness often leads to general immune deficiency, which also is connected often to simultaneous lymphadenopathy.

Silica (converted inside the body to a form of a salt of silicic acid known as silicate orologosilicate) has a fundamental effect on connective tissue weakness and its repercussions. It does not matter this way whether the causes relate to genetic or geriatric reasons or to silica deficiency, as these causes can be improved in like manner.

As human tissue essentially consists of a system of colloids, colloidal solutions of silica, such as silica gel, are particularly suitable for the treatment of connective tissue weakness. A long-term treatment course should be undertaken with daily administration of one to two tablespoons, given pure or administered diluted with water.

In the following, five cases are described in greater detail. All five patients undertook a treatment course of three months with daily two tablespoons of silica gel, according to taste taken pure, or diluted with water.

Patients One to Five

Patient 1: R. K., female, 36 years

Clinical Picture: This patient type's outer appearance already reveals typical connective tissue weakness. She is predisposed to frequent sprains and strains, complains about back pain (caused by weakness of posture), brittle nails, and thin, difficult to manage, hair. Also varicose veins and abnormal proneness for infections of the respiratory tracts exists.

Diagnosis: Inherent constitutional connective tissue weakness.

Therapy: Two tablespoons silica daily for three months.

Pathology: As expected, in the first weeks no noticeable effect results. After six weeks the patient reports that her nails have become sturdier and her hair stronger. During the subsequent treatment course this effect is enhanced, back pain and varicose veins recede, there are no further sprains or strains, even when she walks for protracted periods.

Evaluation: Good therapeutic efficacy.

Patient 2: A. D., female, 27 years

Clinical Picture: The patient complains about chronic digestive and abdominal ailments that can be referred to the prolapse of the intestines. Added to this are first indications of varicose veins, accelerated hair loss and abnormal tendency to sprains and strains especially after prolonged physical exertion.

Diagnosis: Inherent constitutional connective tissue weakness.

Therapy: Two tablespoons silica daily regular supplementation for three months.

Pathology: It takes approximately four weeks until the patient reports a first obvious improvement in hair loss and her digestive complaints. During further progress these effects stabilize and the abdominal pains alleviate. Sprains and strains

following exertions appear only seldom now, the slight tendency to varicose veins has remitted.
Evaluation: Good therapeutic efficacy.

Patient 3: M. B., male, 47 years
Clinical Picture: The patient reports foremost considerable affliction in the joints up to frequent sprains, strains and overstretching even during light physical exertion. He also suffers from weakness of the abdominal wall to the extent of having already undergone two operations for abdominal hernia.

Diagnosis: Inherent constitutional connective tissue weakness.
Therapy: Two tablespoons silica daily regular supplementation for three months.
Pathology: As the patient didn't suffer from acute distress, no direct effects as such were expected. The effect of therapy on the frequency of strains, sprains, and overstretching as the most conspicuous results of the connective tissue weakness was primarily evaluated. In doing so a significant improvement could be achieved, which the patient felt particularly comforting. After the conclusion of therapy the tendency toward such complaints no longer existed. Even the abdominal wall became tauter.

Evaluation: Good therapeutic efficacy.

Patient 4: A. H., female, 43 years
Clinical Picture: The patient complained about developing varicose veins, slack abdominal walls and puffed up skin, but partially also spontaneously, to sprains that heal only slowly during unaccustomed physical exertion. Occasionally rheumatic pains occur around the joints. Nails are often brittle and cracked. Especially conspicuous are the antebrachium veins clearly erupting under the skin.

Diagnosis: Inherent constitutional connective tissue weakness.

Therapy: Two tablespoons silica daily regular supplementation for three months.

Pathology: Initially therapy positively affects skin and nails. During further progress varicose veins clearly recede, and the cosmetically very irritating erupting antebrachium veins are positively influenced. Finally therapy also succeeds in totally eliminating the abnormal tendency to sprains and rheumatic pains.

Evaluation: Good therapeutic efficacy.

Patient 5: P. G., male, 20 years

Clinical Picture: The willowy, tall and lanky young man with a very thin head of hair already suffered from faulty posture, abnormal tendency to sprains, overstretching and infections of the upper respiratory tracts in early childhood. For some time now, increased back pain, obvious slackness of the abdominal wall and connected chronically sluggish bowels complete this picture.

Diagnosis: Inherent constitutional connective tissue weakness.

Therapy: Two tablespoons silica daily regular supplementation for three months.

Pathology: The patient reports, after only a few days, of evident lessening of back pain. Bowel movements are achieved with problem-free regularity. During further therapeutic progress a discernible erectness of posture and firming of abdominal wall is gained. Hair again appears stronger and the tendency to spraining and straining subsides.

Evaluation: Good therapeutic efficacy.

Based on the practical background of these five cases silica gel can be recommended for long term therapy of connective tissue weakness.

Lymphatic Diathesis – Lymphadenopathy – Strengthening the Immune System

The immune system enables the body to cope with harmful intrusions and injurious influences. In this defense system the connective tissue plays a significant role, particularly the reticular connective tissue of the spleen and the lymphatic system.

Through silica, a clear increase of the reticular-endothelial (RES) connective tissue cells is achieved and by that an increase in antibodies (lymphocytes, phagocytes). Silica simultaneously normalizes and strengthens the functions of the entire lymphatic system. This becomes particularly noticeable when a (usually congenital) deficiency of this system exists. Then there is a tendency to frequent swellings of the lymph nodes, an abnormal susceptibility to infection, and general or nervous fitness deterioration.

The stimulation of the immune function is not limited to prevention of colds and other simple infections, of course, or the removal of lymphatic system disturbance, which is known as lymphatic diathesis or lymphadenopathy. The immune defense functions of the connective tissue contribute to the healing process of practically all disorders.

The mobilization of the immune function with silica usually has a positive effect on the pathological process. With increasing environmental organ pollution, it becomes more obvious that silica helps to lighten the ecological burden of the living body. Silica stimulates the detoxified immune response organs.

Satisfactory therapeutic results only can be expected in lymphatic and general immune deficiency following prolonged therapy. In this field study two lymphatic patients received three to four months daily one to two tablespoons regular

111

silica supplementation. In one case study, treated for six weeks only, no notable effects occurred.

Patients Six to Eight

Patient 6: T. S., female, 24 years

Clinical Picture: The patient appears pale. Her very fine, sensitive skin is puffy. Since earliest childhood she tends to abnormal, frequent respiratory tract infections that are accompanied by persistent swellings of the cervical lymph glands. Though the tonsils were removed early in childhood no notable improvement followed.

Diagnosis: Lymphadenopathy

Therapy: One tablespoon silica daily regular supplementation for four months.

Pathology: Within six weeks the patient again suffers a heavy cold with strong swellings of the lymph nodes. In contrast to her history, the swellings definitely retreat quicker and finally retract completely. During further progress, the therapy also proves beneficial to the skin's puffy appearance. Renewed infection that, following earlier history, was to be expected during therapy, did not recur.

Evaluation: Good therapeutic efficacy.

Patient 7: M. H., male, 31 years

Clinical Picture: The patient reports that since boyhood he often suffered from flu infections that ran a difficult course and were regularly accompanied by lymph node tumescence. Lately increasingly metabolic malfunction manifested and the skin became increasingly drier.

Diagnosis: Neurolymphadenopathy

Therapy: Two tablespoons silica daily regular supplementation for 1.5 months.

Pathology: Within the first six weeks the patient reports no meaningful results and therefore ends therapy

on his own. Given sufficiently prolonged therapy a positive therapeutic result probably would
have been possible.

Evaluation: Without therapeutic effect.

Patient 8: H. S., male, 26 years

Clinical Picture: The patient has long been suffering from frequently recurring tumescence of the cervical and subaxillary
lymph nodes. The causes cannot be accurately determined. It
appears however that colds often play a role. Recently there
appears a further tendency to allergic skin reactions that is
repeatedly accompanied by swollen lymph nodes.

Diagnosis: Lymphatic/allergic diathesis

Therapy: One tablespoon silica daily regular supplementation for three months.

Pathology: At the commencement of therapy existing
lymph node tumescence recesses completely
within three weeks. During further progress of
therapy no renewed glandular enlargement can
be observed. As a result no infectious disease
occurs. Still, initially there are occasionally
acute allergic skin manifestations that receive
extra treatment with silica (applied undiluted
three times daily). On conclusion of therapy
these allergic symptoms, too, have vanished.

Evaluation: Very good therapeutic efficacy.

The result of these three cases of the field study verify that
even decades-old lymphatic ailments can be healed through
silica, as long as therapy is consistently followed and continued long enough.

Gastrointestinal Disorders

In the gastrointestinal tract, silica evolves a threefold influence: suppression of infection, natural disinfection and
(similar to organic vegetal charcoal tablets) resorption of

113

gases and toxins. These specific effects are supported by the silica-caused stimulation of the immune system. Silica gel recommends itself for root therapy of inflammations, infections and ulcers of the gastrointestinal tract, variously caused diarrhea, heartburn, acid indigestion, flatulence and for immediate help in poisonings. It is well suited as a home remedy for the prevention and treatment of digestive disturbances and gastrointestinal infections (also while travelling). As silica restores healthy conditions in the gastrointestinal tract, it may also prove beneficial in constipation and intestinal irritation that have arisen from the common misuse of laxatives.

The following six cases illuminate the reliable and partially amazingly quick results. For acute gastrointestinal disease, one tablespoon of pure silica gel was initially administered every two hours. After improvement up to complete recuperation, one tablespoon of silica gel diluted in water was given twice daily. In cases of heartburn, silica gel was diluted in peppermint tea. Therapy lasted altogether 14 to 25 days. Chronic gastrointestinal complaints were treated right from the start by using a daily dose of one to two tablespoons, from four weeks to 2.75 months.

Patients Nine to Fourteen
Patient 9: O. M., male, 60 years
Clinical Picture: The patient suffers from frequently recurring stomach ulcers and chronic hyperacidity for 10 years. His physician counsels surgical procedure as apparently the only alternative, which, however, the patient declines.
Diagnosis: Hyperacidity, ventricular ulcers
Therapy: One tablespoon silica gel two times daily regular supplementation for 2.5 months.
Pathology: Already after the first week the patient reports a marked improvement in his problems. During further progress, symptoms consistently abate.

After conclusion of therapy there are no more complaints. X–ray diagnostics prove the complete healing of the ulcers.

Evaluation: Very good therapeutic efficacy.

Patient 10: H. A., male, four years

Clinical Picture: The patient complains of colicky pains in the abdomen with partially strong flatulence and frequent alterations of diarrhea and constipation. The feces often exhibit traces of mucus.

Diagnosis: Colitis mucosa (inflammation of the large intestine)

Therapy: Initially one tablespoon silica gel daily regular supplementation for three months.

Pathology: The acute symptoms with strong flatulence improve so remarkably within only two days that the administered dosage can be lowered to normal values. During the continued course of treatment colic and flatulence noticeably abate. As of the fifth week defecation has normalized. Occasionally minor complaints occur during the remainder of therapy. Generally a clear improvement was achieved.

Evaluation: Good therapeutic efficacy.

Patient 11: C. S., female, 44 years

Clinical Picture: Due to doubled responsibility load of self-employment and family, the patient is under great stress, which affects her stomach. For some years she suffers from chronic stomach complaints, repletion and lack of appetite. X-ray diagnostics also reveal chronic gastritis.

Diagnosis: Chronic gastritis with strong nervous psychic components.

Therapy: Two tablespoons silica gel daily diluted in water regular supplementation for five weeks. Supplementary autogenous training (endogenous exercise) is prescribed.

Pathology: The patient finds no leisure time to consistently follow autogenous training (endogenous exercise) so that no effect can be expected from exercise. Silica gel, too, achieves only a slight improvement over the five week period. The patient stops therapy.

Evaluation: Moderate therapeutic effect resultant from strong nervous, psychological conditions.

Patient 12: S. F., female, 31 years

Clinical Picture: For months the patient suffers from strong heartburn. The performed desmoid test shows stomach hyperacidity. The cause cannot be definitely diagnosed. Most probably there is a connection to incorrect dietary habits.

Diagnosis: Hyperacidity with suspicion of chronic stomach hypersensitivity.

Therapy: One tablespoon silica gel daily at noon in peppermint tea regular supplementation for 1.5 months.

Pathology: The heartburn abruptly subsides already on the third treatment day. The accompanying vague digestive problems remain for some time. After approximately one month the patient reports general freedom from symptoms. The desmoid test shows nearly normal stomach acid levels at the conclusion of therapy.

Evaluation: Good therapeutic efficacy.

Patient 13: P. K., male, 53 years

Clinical Picture: The patient contracted a serious intestinal infection during his holidays some months prior. Though this is completely healed, according to orthodox medical therapy of his regular physician, he still suffers from diarrhea and strong digestive disorders that so far have not responded to therapy.

Diagnosis: Neglected gastroenteritis.

Therapy: One tablespoon silica gel two times daily for five weeks.

Pathology: At first, the patient presumes that silicic acid worsens his ailment. Whether this is a kind of "at first" therapeutic reaction due to the stimulation of the immune system cannot be determined accurately enough. Yet, after 16 days he reports a noticeable improvement of his digestive complaints and abatement of the diarrhea. This result cannot be markedly improved upon until the termination of therapy.

Evaluation: Satisfactory therapeutic efficacy.

Patient 14: S. U., female, 41 years

Clinical Picture: The patient often suffers from strong, partially diet-related flatulence and irregular bowel movements with a tendency to constipation. Symbiotic bacteria control therapy, "tentatively" prescribed, brings no noticeable improvement. Linseed therapy could not satisfactorily improve sluggishness of the bowels.

Diagnosis: Meteorism with constipation

Therapy: One tablespoon silica gel two times daily regular supplementation for six weeks.

Pathology: Already from the second week, a notable alleviation of flatulence occurs. During the further treatment period the patient reports that her bowel movements slowly normalize. After conclusion of therapy, flatulence occurs only seldom. Emptying of the bowels succeeds almost regularly every day.

Evaluation: Good therapeutic efficacy.

Kidney, Bladder and Women's Disorders

Within the framework of this field study, the particular efficacy of silica gel in urological and gynaecological diseases was not tested. Therefore no sample test cases can be cited.

Still, good therapeutic results from silicic acid treatment in such cases have been reported in the professional literature.

The influence of silica gel on urinary organs shows in increased diuresis, which researcher Breitenstein found to be up to 37 percent. Silica gel is also used as a prophylaxis against kidney stone colic. Inflammation of the kidneys, conducting urinary tracts, and in particular, the urinary bladder respond well to the anti-inflammatory, biologically disinfectant effect of silicic acid.

Additionally, silica gel increases urination by up to 37 percent so that the diseased urinary organs are thoroughly flushed. In cases of simple cystitis (inflammation of the bladder) this usually is sufficient for treatment. However, in cases of kidney disease, other biological medicines (if need be also antibiotics) must be given. For basic therapy, however, silica gel is always recommended. This is especially so due to silica's immune system enhancing effect.

Different practical axperiences show that silicic acid prevents kidney stones. So it should be prescribed as an additional (preventive) treatment course in cases of known predisposition or as a follow-up treatment course (prevention of recurrence after kidney stone removal).

In gynaecological problems, silica gel is recommended mainly for its strong anti-inflammatory effect in cases of mastitis, i.e., inflammation of the mammary glands (also during the lying-in period). External focal application should preferably be supplemented daily with ingestion of one to two tablespoons of silicic acid. This combined therapy usually brings faster results.

Other gynaecological uses, which, however, always require professional treatment control, are vaginal discharges, abscesses and ulcerations (ulcers, furuncles, boils, sores, craters) in the genital area and around the mouth of the womb. In such cases, on the advice of the therapist, silica gel often lends itself to tamponade therapy, i.e., tampons saturated with silica gel. Supplementary inner treatment is always recommendable. This activates the body's immune powers and plays a role in healing.

Even in cases of urogenital tract diseases when silica gel is not always enough for exclusive therapy, it represents an important additional treatment support for the biological oriented professional. It often noticeably shortens the progress of a disease.

Arterial Sclerosis and Secondary Ailments in Old Age
Hardening and narrowing of the arteries is so widespread nowadays, it has taken on epidemic proportions. It often notably decreases life expectancy and the quality of life. There are practically no citizens of the industrial nations on the other side of sixty years of age who do not show at least a sclerosis of the main arteries, the aortas. More often, however, greater areas of the arterial network are affected. Not seldom, the first arteriosclerotic changes occur already during the third or fourth decade of life. Beyond the fiftieth year of life, they most often represent the cause of premature aging.

Arteriosclerosis is unpleasant enough. Even more feared, however, are its secondary or resultant conditions, most particularly heart attack and stroke. High blood pressure, too, is connected to arteriosclerosis. On the one hand, it promotes vascular diseases; on the other hand, it is worsened by the constriction and hardening of the blood vessels.

The causes of this disease of civilization, arteriosclerosis, are not fully known even today. Beyond doubt though, it

119

can be said that incorrect nutrition, a high fat and calorie-rich diet, stress and a generally unhealthy lifestyle play a central role in its establishment. Genetic factors correspondingly lose in importance because genetic predisposition can be held in check with a reasonable lifestyle. Therapy for existing vascular changes is problematic. Until recently, it was held that existing arterial damages could not be reversed. Meanwhile certain approaches, including juice fasting and/or chelation therapy, offer a kind of scrubbing out of the arteries. It is nonetheless the better course to prevent arteriosclerosis in the first place or to at least treat it vigorously in its early stages. In this, the element silicon plays a decisive role. This is confirmed by the following 14 cases. The effect of silicic acid first shows its favorable influence on the elastic connective tissue of the arterial walls. Then there is the partial or complete reversal of the deswelling of the intima: the inner vascular wall. This makes the arteries elastic again. Blood flow increases and high blood pressure is lowered. Silica gel therefore achieves a lessening of arteriosclerotic complaints, favorably influences their causes and prevents the feared secondary diseases. Practical experience gained with the following 14 patients agrees with other authors of professional papers.

Patients 15 to 28

Patient 15: M. T., female, 76 years
Clinical Picture: The patient suffers from chronically cold, pallid lower extremities. After longer periods of walking, painful calves are added to this picture. In addition, she experiences vertigo, impaired memory, frequent headaches and moderately higher blood pressure.
Diagnosis: Arteriosclerosis with hypertension.
Therapy: One tablespoon of silica gel daily regular supplementation for three months.
Pathology: There is no notable effect within the first four

weeks. After that the patient reports that the incidences of vertigo and headaches have lessened. A slight lowering of blood pressure can be measured. Toward the end of therapy, all complaints have lessened. Blood pressure is nearly normal.

Evaluation: Satisfactory therapeutic efficacy.

Patient 16: F. P., male, 68 years

Clinical Picture: General debility, vertigo, tinnitus, headaches, forgetfulness and a tendency to depression is the disease syndrome of this patient.

Diagnosis: Cerebral arteriosclerosis

Therapy: One tablespoon silica gel two times daily regular supplementation for 2.75 months.

Pathology: Though the patient soon reports slight improvements of circulatory disturbances, this effect cannot be further enhanced. It may be due to the irregular way the patient, not following the therapeutic instructions, supplements with silica gel.

Evaluation: Moderate therapeutic efficacy.

Patient 17: I. O., female, 63 years

Clinical Picture: This patient experiences mainly chronic congestion in the head, vertigo, and sleep disturbances. Additionally, there are chronically cold feet and increased blood pressure.

Diagnosis: Arteriosclerosis with hypertension.

Therapy: One tablespoon silica gel two times daily regular supplementation for two months.

Pathology: First there is an improvement of the blood flow through the lower extremities. Incidence of vertigo lessen. After approximately one month the congestion of the head noticeably recedes. Sleep pattern and blood pressure normalize. In the further course of the treatment plan these effects stabilize and after conclusion of therapy there remain only light complaints.

Evaluation: Good therapeutic efficacy.

Patient 18: A. S., female, 59 years

Clinical Picture: For some time now, this patient suffers from clearly decreasing vitality that is complicated by vertigo, congestion of the head, forgetfulness and dyspnea (shortness of breath) connected to bodily exertion. Blood pressure is slightly increased.

Diagnosis: Early arteriosclerosis

Therapy: One tablespoon silica gel daily regular supplementation for 1.75 months.

Pathology: Within a few short days the patient reports lessening of vertigo. After that the diminishment of symptoms progressed rapidly. The former vitality returns. Following therapy there are practically no complaints. Blood pressure is in the upper normal range.

Evaluation: Very good therapeutic efficacy.

Patient 19: D. M., female, 69 years

Clinical Picture: The patient seems weepy, complains of chronic headaches, tinnitus (buzzing of the ears) and a constant feeling of cold throughout her body. Her relatives report that she's become increasingly distrustful of others recently and sleeps poorly.

Diagnosis: Advanced arteriosclerosis.

Therapy: One tablespoon silica gel two times daily regular supplementation for 2.3 months.

Pathology: The patient proves to be difficult to talk with. She transfers her distrust to the therapist and believes that no one can help her. This causes unreliable administration of silica gel. She also doesn't regularly attend examinations. She reports no effects. Finally she refuses continuation of therapy before any noticeable effect can be achieved.

Evaluation: No therapeutic effect.

Patient 20: G. H., male, 56 years

Clinical Picture: The patient generally feels good. For some time now he experiences that his legs fall asleep, tingle unpleasantly, or hurt following longer exertions. His memory has slowly deteriorated.

Diagnosis: Beginning arteriosclerosis.

Therapy: One tablespoon silica gel daily regular supplementation for nine weeks.

Pathology: The patient tends to self-observation. Probably for this reason he reports slight improvements already after three days (possibly imaginary). During the further treatment course the complaints, however, quickly abate. After therapy the legs still fall asleep at times, however, tingling and pain do not recur and memory is improved.

Evaluation: Good therapeutic efficacy.

Patient 21: K. N., male, 70 years

Clinical Picture: The patient, formerly a heavy smoker, fears for this reason that circulatory disturbances in the legs will sooner or later lead to a necessity of amputation. Otherwise he still feels well and actively participates in life.

Diagnosis: Arteriosclerosis in both legs.

Therapy: One tablespoon silica gel two times daily regular supplementation for four months.

Pathology: A long time passes before the first slight effect is noticeable. After that improvements of blood flow through both legs are rapid and after three months complaints are reduced too after longer or strenuous exertion. Preventively, therapy is continued for another month without any regression or recurrence.

Evaluation: Good therapeutic efficacy.

Patient 22: R. L., female, 67 years

Clinical Picture: The patient suffers from heavy circulatory disorder of her extremities, vertigo, frequent headaches and moderately increased blood pressure.

Diagnosis: Arteriosclerosis.

Therapy: One tablespoon silica gel two times daily regular supplementation for 2.4 months.

Pathology: After approximately 3 weeks the patient reports lessening of the headaches. Blood pressure shows improvement. During the further treatment course, headaches and vertigo lessen notably. Circulatory disturbances of the extremities are not influenced to the same degree.

Evaluation: Satisfactory therapeutic efficacy.

Patient 23: H. Z., male, 64 years

Clinical Picture: Until his retirement two years earlier, this patient "never had time to get sick." Now he suffers heart pain, shortness of breath, chronically cold limbs and buzzing of the ears. No organic heart trouble is found. Blood pressure is generally normal.

Diagnosis: Light arteriosclerosis with psychological-nervous complaints (retirement shock)

Therapy: One tablespoon silica gel two times daily regular supplementation for two months.

Pathology: As psychological-nervous factors play an important role, prognosis seems poor from the beginning. Only after the first month the patient reports a slight improvement in his tinnitus. During the further treatment course, blood circulation in the limbs improves somewhat. Otherwise the therapy does little.

Evaluation: Moderate therapeutic efficacy.

Patient 24: B. W., female, 68 years
Clinical Picture: The patient reports sleep disturbances, vertigo and frequent congestion of the head. She also complains of light pains in her calves following prolonged walking.

Diagnosis: Arteriosclerosis.
Therapy: One tablespoon silica gel daily regular supplementation for 1.5 months.
Pathology: Vertigo and congestion of the head subside after three weeks. Sleep is improved. Pain in the calves is not much influenced. Overall the patient is satisfied with the results.
Evaluation: Satisfactory therapeutic efficacy.

Patient 25: R. A., male, 72 years
Clinical Picture: Chronically cold, often numb, pale-bluish extremities are in the foreground of the clinical picture. Occasionally there is vertigo with tinnitus and dysopia (visual disturbances). Blood pressure is moderately increased.

Diagnosis: Arteriosclerosis.
Therapy: One tablespoon silica gel daily regular supplementation for three months.
Pathology: At first the patient reports slight warming of the hands. After that, the circulation of the limbs is clearly improved. After conclusion of the therapy, vertigo and its accompanying complaints occur hardly at all.
Evaluation: Satisfactory therapeutic efficacy.

Patient 26: L. F., male, 64 years
Clinical Picture: The patient suffers from strong memory weakness. Often there are additional vertigo attacks. Besides, he often feels cold at normal temperatures.

Diagnosis: Cerebral sclerosis.

Therapy: Two tablespoons silica gel daily regular supplementation for 2.66 months.

Pathology: After two weeks the vertigo is clearly improved. The feeling of cold abates. During the course of further treatment memory power increased notably and after conclusion of therapy all complaints are almost completely gone.

Evaluation: Good therapeutic efficacy.

Patient 27: H. D., female, 69 years

Clinical Picture: The patient complains mostly of vertigo, memory and concentration problems and cold feet. Additionally, she is often depressed and has trouble sleeping.

Diagnosis: Light arteriosclerosis.

Therapy: One tablespoon silica gel daily regular supplementation for three months.

Pathology: After a few days, the vertigo abates. From the third week, circulation of the legs is noticeably improved. During the course of further treatment, memory and concentration are normalized. After therapy there are no more ailments.

Evaluation: Very good therapeutic efficacy.

Patient 28: V. B., female, 66 years

Clinical Picture: The patient suffers from unstable hypertension. For some time frequent vertigo and numb limbs occur. Sometimes there are heart and calf pains when walking.

Diagnosis: Arteriosclerosis with changeable hypertension.

Therapy: One tablespoon silica gel daily regular supplementation for 2.3 months.

Pathology: Heart and calf pains respond well to therapy. After that it takes some time before the vertigo and the numb limbs improve. The ailments cannot be completely remedied.

Evaluation: Satisfactory therapeutic efficacy.

Based on this practical experience, arteriosclerosis shows as a most important indication of silica gel. Additionally, silicic acid generally lends itself well for prevention and therapy in geriatrics. Aging symptoms occur due to the loss of water in the tissues (dehydration) and the deswelling of the proteins with increased protein denaturing. Sufficient water binding and protein swelling set important preconditions for all plasma life processes. Silica gel improves water binding and protein swelling again and so prevents premature aging or improves aging symptoms that occur too soon. Silica gel, of course, cannot prevent the natural process of aging. It nonetheless plays an important role in slowing down aging and bringing the aging mechanism within currently accepted values. In this, it supports today's modern human being to attain the life expectancy that is pre-programmed by nature. It does this so that stronger complaints of aging do not notably reduce the quality of life.

Bronchial Catarrh – Bronchitis – Lung Diseases

Silica occurs in abundance in the connective tissue of the lungs that contains very many elastic fibers. This shows its importance for this vital organic system. With increasing age, sufficient supply of silicic acid for the respiratory system becomes ever more important. On the one hand, the elasticity of the lung decreases due to aging (this can lead to lung emphysema). On the other hand, tissues that can slow down or revert this aging process, become poor in silica.

Therapy with silica gel is therefore also best for the maintenance and strengthening of the respiratory system following the midpoint in life. Silicic acid is of particular importance in cases of lung tuberculosis. In this disease there is a lack of silica of up to 50 percent in the lung tissues. This must be balanced through long term therapy with this trace element. Simultaneously, silica gel assists in accelerating the encapsulation and demarcation of the tubercular foci.

Silica gel also meaningfully supplements therapy in other lung diseases.

Within the framework of this field study, silica gel was tested for its efficacy also in bronchial catarrh and bronchitis. The focus was on intractable or obstinate bronchial ailments that could not be influenced satisfactorily by other means. In such cases, silica gel acts as an anti-inflammatory and strengthens the immune system. It alleviates coughing and is expectorant. This provides a versatile therapy encompassing many primary causes and preventing secondary diseases of the lungs.

Patients 29 to 37

Patient 29: H. O., male, 59 years
Clinical Picture: Since a cold of approximately eight months ago, the patient suffers from an obstinate cough. Especially in the mornings much mucous is thrown out. Body temperature is not increased.

Diagnosis: Neglected bronchial catarrh.
Therapy: One tablespoon silica gel two times daily regular supplementation for 1.25 months.
Pathology: Already after one week the patient reports a first alleviation of his cough. During the further course of therapy, all symptoms dissipate completely. After approximately five weeks, the patient can be released as having been completely healed.
Evaluation: Very good therapeutic efficacy.

Patient 30: F. M., male, 37 years
Clinical Picture: The patient smokes a lot. For years he has suffered from typical smoker's cough, especially in the mornings.

Diagnosis: Chronic bronchial catarrh through nicotine abuse.
Therapy: One tablespoon silica gel two times daily regu-

lar supplementation for 1.5 months. No smoking allowed.

Pathology: The patient cannot tolerate going without nicotine for too long. Instead he increases now and then the prescribed dosage up to five tablespoons (which is tolerated well). His smoker's catarrh is only slightly improved due to his continued nicotine consumption.

Evaluation: Moderate therapeutic efficacy.

Patient 31: A. W., female, 55 years
Clinical Picture: The patient continues to suffer after enduring a heavy, purulent bronchitis that was treated with antibiotics. There still is strong coughing and pain under the breastbone.
Diagnosis: Chronic bronchitis.
Therapy: One tablespoon silica gel two times daily regular supplementation for two months.
Pathology: During the first three weeks there is no noticeable improvement. After that, the coughing is more seldom and softer. This effect increases. After the conclusion of therapy the patient coughs only occasionally.
Evaluation: Good therapeutic efficacy.

Patient 32: C. S., female, 35 years
Clinical Picture: The patient complains of frequent but light coughing with thick-transparent sputum that is difficult to expel.
Diagnosis: Dry, neglected bronchial catarrh.
Therapy: One tablespoon silica gel daily regular supplementation for three to five days.
Pathology: The patient responds quickly to therapy with a clearly decreased cough. Shortly after that she reports that the sputum can be expelled with greater ease during coughing. Though some complaints remain, she breaks off therapy early.
Evaluation: Satisfactory therapeutic efficacy.

Patient 33: M. K., female, 65 years
Clinical Picture: Moderate nicotine consumption of this patient so far has hindered the healing of a heavy, neglected bronchitis that she's had for months. It has also caused shortness of breath.

Diagnosis: Chronic bronchitis with respiratory distress.

Therapy: One tablespoon silica gel two times daily regular supplementation for two to five months.

Pathology: The cough continues unabated for approximately four weeks. Then there is a slow improvement despite continued nicotine abuse. Expectoration of mucus increases and breathing is eased. After the conclusion of therapy there is still a light cough because of nicotine consumption.

Evaluation: Satisfactory therapeutic efficacy.

Patient 34: P. S., male, 39 years
Clinical Picture: The patient suffers during treatment from another ailment – an acute infection with strong cough and mild fever.

Diagnosis: Acute bronchial catarrh.

Therapy: One tablespoon silica gel two times daily regular supplementation for three weeks.

Pathology: The cough improves on the third day. Body temperature normalizes after five days. During further treatment, the cough is completely healed.

Evaluation: Good therapeutic efficacy.

Patient 35: T. R., female, 40 years
Clinical Picture: The patient, after a neglected cold, suffers from mucus congestion of the bronchi with moderate coughing.

Diagnosis: Neglected bronchial catarrh.

Therapy: One tablespoon silica gel daily regular supplementation for four weeks.

Pathology: During the second week coughing is temporarily increased. This, simultaneously, leads to greater discharge of mucus. After that, the catarrh abates except for minor residual complaints.

Evaluation: Satisfactory therapeutic efficacy.

Patient 36: E. G., male, 51 years

Clinical Picture: The patient complains of chronic, light coughing with greenish phlegm with a light fever. He sometimes feels a stitch in the side during coughing.

Diagnosis: Chronic bronchitis.

Therapy: One tablespoon silica gel two times daily regular supplementation for 1.8 months.

Pathology: Initially the phlegm turns whitish and the stitch in the side disappears. During the course of treatment, the coughing noticeably abates but cannot be completely cleared by the end of therapy.

Evaluation: Satisfactory therapeutic efficacy.

Patient 37: L. H., male, 52 years

Clinical Picture: After an accident with caustic gases, the patient suffers from bronchial irritation with coughing and mucilaginous congestion.

Diagnosis: Chronic bronchial catarrh.

Therapy: One tablespoon silica gel two times daily regular supplementation for two months.

Pathology: The effect is slow in coming with a slowly abating cough and increased expectoration. During the course of further treatment, the problems visibly abate. After the conclusion of therapy only a light, infrequent cough remains.

Evaluation: Good therapeutic efficacy.

The previous nine cases show the good effect of silica gel on acute or chronic catarrh of the bronchi. Regardless of causes, convincing therapeutic results are achieved. Only in one case is this unsatisfactory, due to the patient's continued smoking.

Colds, Coughs and Catarrh of Throat and Larynx
The good, anti-inflammatory, immune system activating effect of silica gel is recommended for therapy of acute and chronic inflammations of the upper respiratory tract. Gargling and rinsing can be supplemented and, depending on need, with ingestion. This seems advisable especially in cases of chronic diseases that can influence the causes in an encompassing manner.

Patients 38 to 51
Patient 38: E. P., male, 38 years
Clinical Picture: The patient suffers from a chronically blocked nose and dry nasal membranes for years.
Diagnosis: Chronic head cold (rhinitis sicca).
Therapy: One teaspoon silica gel sniffed up diluted with two parts of water for seven weeks.
Pathology: The patient finds the eased nose breathing, that sets in after just a few days, especially agreeable. Unfortunately the dry nasal membranes are not completely improved. However, they no longer cause discomfort
Evaluation: Satisfactory therapeutic efficacy.

Patient 39: A. O., female, 67 years
Clinical Picture: Patient alternately suffers from a dry nose with difficult breathing and attacks of strong nasal secretion.
Diagnosis: Head cold (nervous vasomotor rhinitis).
Therapy: One teaspoon silica gel sniffed up three times daily diluted with two parts water regular for four weeks.
Pathology: The patient soon reports that the dryness of nose and respiration eases. The symptoms can-

not be totally removed. The attacks of secretion are not influenced.

Evaluation: Moderate therapeutic efficacy.

Patient 40: C. R., female, 45 years

Clinical Picture: The patient undergoes treatment for another ailment and suffers an acute cold during that time.

Diagnosis: Acute infectious rhinitis.

Therapy: Six times daily one teaspoon silica gel sniffed up undiluted for a total of three days. Then for post-treatment, 14 days of three times daily one teaspoon of silica gel sniffed up diluted with water 1:2.

Pathology: The cold responds immediately well to therapy. The secretion abates and the nasal respiration becomes more free. As a slight dryness is in the nose after three days, treatment for another two weeks is continued with a reduced dosage.

Evaluation: Very good therapeutic efficacy.

Patient 41: H. N., female, 60 years

Clinical Picture: Following misuse of mucous membrane deswelling nose sprays, the patient suffers from dry nasal mucosa with bark and mucosa loss.

Diagnosis: Atrophying rhinitis (turning into ozaena).

Therapy: Five times one teaspoon silica gel sniffed up daily with two parts water for 2.3 months.

Pathology: The effect shows after ten days. During the further treatment course improvement continues at a slow pace. After conclusion of therapy the nasal mucosa is largely normalized.

Evaluation: Good therapeutic efficacy.

Patient 42: K. U., male, 39 years

Clinical Picture: The patient suffers from a chronically furry voice. Sometimes this is aggravated by pain in the larynx.

The symptoms show breathing through the mouth.

Diagnosis: Chronic laryngitis.

Therapy: Three times daily gargling with one tablespoon silica gel in a dilution of three times as much water. Also ingestion of one tablespoon silica gel for a total period of six weeks.

Pathology: In the first three weeks the hoarseness recedes only haltingly. After that, improvements accelerate and there is no further pain. After therapy there is only occasional hoarseness.

Evaluation: Satisfactory therapeutic efficacy.

Patient 43: N. Z., female, 56 years

Clinical Picture: The patient suffers from persistent scratching of the throat; the pharynx is dry and reddened.

Diagnosis: Chronic pharyngeal catarrh.

Therapy: Four times daily gargling with one tablespoon silica gel diluted with three tablespoons of water for 1.25 months.

Pathology: The patient reports an improvement of her scratchy throat already on the second day. After that, the effect becomes even stronger. After therapy there are no more complaints. The pharynx is still a little dry though.

Evaluation: Good therapeutic efficacy.

Patient 44: P. S., male, 61 years

Clinical Picture: After a heavy cold, the patient is suffering from coughing and hoarseness for months. The pharynx is moderately reddened.

Diagnosis: Pharyngeal-laryngeal catarrh with coughing.

Therapy: Two times daily gargling with one tablespoon silica gel diluted with three parts (three tablespoons) of water. Internal ingestion of two times daily one tablespoon. Treatment course of 1.66 months altogether.

Pathology: As a first sign, the cough improves. The amount of phlegm increases. After that all symptoms visibly recede. At the end of therapy there are no more complaints.

Evaluation: Very good therapeutic efficacy.

Patient 45: R. R., female, 54 years

Clinical Picture: The patient complains of a sore throat and chronic cough lasting several weeks. Initially, there was also a runny nose that meanwhile has cleared up.

Diagnosis: Neglected Pharyngeal-laryngeal bronchial catarrh (bronchitis).

Therapy: Three times daily gargling with one tablespoon silica gel diluted with three parts water. Internal ingestion two times daily one tablespoon. Treatment period of four weeks altogether.

Pathology: The cough improves quickly and markedly. The pain continues unabated for some time and only subsides toward the end of treatment. The cough is almost completely healed.

Evaluation: Satisfactory therapeutic efficacy.

Patient 46: H. M., male, 72 years

Clinical Picture: The patient suffers from chronic laryngitis and cough resultant from a chronic infection.

Diagnosis: Chronic laryngitis and bronchitis.

Therapy: Two times daily gargling with one tablespoon silica gel diluted with three parts of water. Internal ingestion two times one tablespoon. Treatment period of seven weeks altogether.

Pathology: After 11 days the patient reports improvement of cough and laryngitis. This result stabilizes. Still, a total healing does not occur until the end of the therapy period.

Evaluation: Satisfactory therapeutic efficacy.

Patient 47: L. W., female, 58 years
Clinical Picture: The patient complains of throat and pharynx pain (strong larynx reddening) and a moderate cough.
Diagnosis: Acute pharyngitis.
Therapy: Four times daily gargling with one tablespoon silica gel diluted with three parts water for 24 days.
Pathology: First improvements occur quickly and continue. After the conclusion of therapy there are no more complaints.
Evaluation: Very good therapeutic efficacy.

Patient 48: G. S., male, 67 years
Clinical Picture: The patient suffers from chronic pain and dryness in the areas of throat and pharynx for years.
Diagnosis: Chronic pharyngitis.
Therapy: Three times daily gargling with one tablespoon silica gel diluted with three parts water. Internal ingestion of one tablespoon silica gel. Total treatment period lasts two months.
Pathology: There is a slight improvement within the first three weeks. The pace of healing accelerates after that and then stabilizes. The dryness of throat cannot be totally overcome.
Evaluation: Satisfactory therapeutic efficacy.

Patient 49: C. M., female, 43 years
Clinical Picture: Following a cold, the patient, a heavy smoker, suffers from chronic laryngitis and a light cough for some months.
Diagnosis: Neglected laryngitis with coughing.
Therapy: Two times daily gargling with one tablespoon silica gel diluted with three parts water. Internal ingestion of one tablespoon silica gel two times daily. Treatment period lasts altogether six weeks.
Pathology: The patient persists in smoking against medical advice and soon smokes as much as ever.

Despite this, her cough completely abates after therapy. The laryngitis is markedly improved.

Evaluation: Satisfactory therapeutic efficacy.

Patient 50: P. A., male, 52 years

Clinical Picture: The patient suffers from blocked nasal passages, burning and scratching sensations in the throat, occasional cough.

Diagnosis: Chronic rhino-pharyngitis.

Therapy: Four times daily one teaspoon silica gel diluted with two parts water sniffed up. Two times daily gargling with one tablespoon diluted with three parts water. Internal ingestion of one tablespoon silica gel daily. Total treatment period lasts six weeks.

Pathology: The patient responds quickly and well to therapy. Pharyngitis and cough noticeably improve with later freeing of the nasal passages. Toward the end of therapy there are hardly any complaints.

Evaluation: Good therapeutic efficacy.

Patient 51: B. V., male, 39 years

Clinical Picture:The patient suffers from chronic laryngitis for months. So far no treatment succeeded.

Diagnosis: Chronic laryngitis.

Therapy: Two times daily gargling with one tablespoon silica gel diluted with three parts water. Internal ingestion of one tablespoon silica gel two times daily. Total treatment period lasts four weeks.

Pathology: Already in the first week there is a slight improvement that quickly intensifies. After therapy there is still sometimes laryngitis if the voice is used intensively. Otherwise, there are no more complaints.

Evaluation: Good therapeutic efficacy.

Stomatitis – Gum Diseases and Tooth Decay Prevention

In diseases of the oral mucosa and the gums silica gel is anti-inflammatory and activates the focal immune system. The functional ability of the tissues improves so much that even cases of acute gum recession respond to therapy. Silica's styptic, hemostatic effect is of help if the picture is complicated by bleeding gums. Silica gel also plays a preventive role in tooth decay. It is thought that silica functions as a "tug" for calcium, i.e., promotes calcium attachment and placement into the teeth so that the teeth can withstand the onslaught of tooth decay better. For all such cases, silicic acid is used as an internal therapeutic. One to two tablespoons are administered daily. In diseases of the mouth and gums a focal rinsing treatment is often sufficient.

The following reports practical experiences with silica gel within the framework of this field study. This study did not test silica toothpaste and/or oral rinse, which might be more suitable to this type of therapy depending on circumstances.

Patients 52 to 60

Patient 52: A. K., female, 55 years

Clinical Picture: The patient suffers from stomatitis with swelling of the pharyngeal lymph nodes, bad mouth odor and early gingivitis (inflammation of the gums).

Diagnosis: Stomatitis and gingivitis.

Therapy: Four times daily mouth rinse with one table-spoon silica gel diluted with three parts water. Treatment period lasts 23 days.

Pathology: Pain abates noticeably within three days. After the conclusion of therapy there is only occasional mouth odor. Otherwise, there are no more complaints.

Evaluation: Good therapeutic efficacy.

Patient 53: K. M., male, 43 years
Clinical Picture: The patient suffers continuously from stomatitis and gingivitis because of nicotine abuse.
Diagnosis: Chronic stomatitis and gingivitis.
Therapy: Four times daily mouth rinse with one table-spoon silica gel diluted with three parts water. Total treatment lasts one month.
Pathology: Though the patient will not stop smoking, there soon is a marked improvement in his condition. Complete healing is impossible under condi-tions of continued nicotine abuse.
Evaluation: Satisfactory therapeutic efficacy.

Patient 54: D. X., female, 54 years
Clinical Picture: Due to insufficient mouth hygiene, the patient suffers from frequently painful infections and ulcers of the oral mucosa.
Diagnosis: Chronic, recurrent stomatitis.
Therapy: Four times daily mouth rinse with one1 table-spoon silica gel diluted with three parts water for 1.3 months.
Pathology: Already on the second day the pain lessens. During the further course of treatment, improvements are slower. At the conclusion of therapy there still are slight residual complaints.
Evaluation: Satisfactory therapeutic efficacy.

Patient 55: T. E., female, 58 years
Clinical Picture: The patient suffers from yellow-whitish covered ulcers on the mucous membrane and the gums.
Diagnosis: Acute stomatitis aphthosa (herpes virus).
Therapy: Four times daily mouth rinse with one table-spoon silica gel diluted in three parts water for a total treatment period of one month.
Pathology: Pain disappears quickly. The mouth becomes drier. After the conclusion of therapy the ulcer-

ations and infections heal completely.

Evaluation: Very good therapeutic efficacy.

Patient 56: O. V., male, 64 years

Clinical Picture: The patient, treated for another ailment, complains of pressure pain from his dentures. His dentist could not eliminate this problem so far.

Diagnosis: Chronic irritation of the mucous membranes.

Therapy: Three times daily mouth rinse with one tablespoon silica gel diluted with three parts water for a total treatment period of three weeks.

Pathology: The areas affected by denture pressure quickly improve. After the conclusion of therapy there are only slight residual problems. The patient wants to continue the silica gel treatment until his dentist can correctly fit the dentures.

Evaluation: Satisfactory therapeutic efficacy.

Patient 57: B. H., male, 48 years

Clinical Picture: The patient suffers from chronic gum recession and frequent gum bleeding.

Diagnosis: Creeping periodontal disease (gum recession).

Therapy: Two times daily mouth rinse with one tablespoon silica gel diluted with three parts water. Mornings and evenings gum massaging with one tablespoon undiluted silica gel each, with a treatment duration of nine weeks.

Pathology: The bleeding stops after a few days. The gums tauten and strengthen again.

Evaluation: Good therapeutic efficacy.

Patient 58: M. T., female, 56 years

Clinical Picture: The patient suffers from chronic gum recession and inflammation with bleeding gums.

Diagnosis: Chronic periodontal disease and gingivitis.

Therapy: Three times daily mouth rinse with one tablespoon silica gel diluted with three parts water. Mornings and nights gum massaging with one tablespoon undiluted silica gel each. Internal ingestion of one tablespoon two times daily for a total treatment period of two months.

Pathology: After two weeks there is no more bleeding. The inflammation improves. After the conclusion of therapy there is no further bleeding or inflammation. The gums tauten.

Evaluation: Very good therapeutic efficacy.

Patient 59: F. D., female, 48 years

Clinical Picture: The very sensitive gums of the patient tend to frequent inflammations and bleeding.

Diagnosis: Genetic predisposition to gum bleeding and gum inflammations.

Therapy: Two times daily gargling with one tablespoon silica gel diluted in three parts water. Mornings and nights gum massaging with each one tablespoon undiluted silica gel. Internal ingestion of one tablespoon silica gel daily. Total treatment period extends over eight weeks.

Pathology: After two weeks the gum bleeding subsides. During further treatment all complaints nearly disappear totally.

Evaluation: Good therapeutic efficacy.

Patient 60: G. A., male, 60 years

Clinical Picture: The patient suffers from gum bleeding and chronic gum recession.

Diagnosis: Chronic periodontal disease with gum bleeding.

Therapy: Four times daily gargling with one tablespoon silica gel each diluted with three parts water. Mornings and evenings gum massaging with each one tablespoon undiluted silica gel for a total treatment period of 2.5 months.

Pathology: After three weeks gum bleeding does not occur any longer. Slowly the gum recession abates. The gums tauten and circulatory blood flow supply improves.
Evaluation: Good therapeutic efficacy.

Skin Diseases and Injuries
Lack of silica often shows first in brittle nails, premature aging, flabby or withered skin and especially in feminine hair loss at any age. Male hair loss, especially hair loss in younger men, more often comes from genetic predisposition or sex hormone factors. These factors, however, in no way invalidate benefits that men can derive from long term silica gel supplementation. For all these reasons, silica gel belongs to the daily care of skin, hair, and nails. Silica gel is recommended also from without, especially in cases of skin irritations, inflammations, reddening, suppurations, allergies, itching, insect bites and sunburn. Silica gel helps heal small skin injuries, excessive foot sweat and wetness between the toes with danger of developing fungi infections, such as athlete's foot.

In all these circumstances, silica gel relieves irritations, works as an anti-inflammatory, is absorbent, cooling, painkilling and eliminates itchiness. Silica gel promotes healing and strengthens the immune system. Ingestion supports external focal uses. The following thirteen cases from the field study describe diseases and injuries of the skin, hair and nails in greater detail.

Patients 61 to 73
Patient 61: E. N., female, 49 years
Clinical Picture: The patient suffers from strong, itchy skin allergies with reddening and blistering (vesication, vesiculation).
Diagnosis: Allergic rashes.

Therapy: Three times daily silica gel undiluted focally applied to affected skin areas for a total treatment period of 18 days.

Pathology: Itching promptly stops. During the further treatment period the reddening and blistering recede.

Evaluation: Very good therapeutic efficacy.

Patient 62: L. B., female, 55 years

Clinical Picture: The patient suffers from wizened, prematurely aged skin and cosmetically unsightly brittle nails.

Diagnosis: Premature skin aging due to connective tissue weakness and deficient silicic acid.

Therapy: Two times daily ingestion of one tablespoon silica gel. Three times undiluted focally applied as facial mask for 10 minutes, then washed off. Total treatment period lasts 2.5 months.

Pathology: The nails become harder, the skin tauter and fresher. This effect becomes increasingly visible.

Evaluation: Good therapeutic efficacy.

Patient 63: H. R., male, 44 years

Clinical Picture: The patient contracted a sunburn, mainly on shoulders, breast and back.

Diagnosis: Sunburn.

Therapy: Two times daily two tablespoons silica gel diluted with three parts water focally applied to affected skin areas for a total treatment period of 14 days.

Pathology: Burning and pain subsides quickly. Within a few days, the sunburn heals completely.

Evaluation: Very good therapeutic efficacy.

Patient 64: J. T., female, 62 years

Clinical Picture: The patient suffers from itchiness of the lower thighs, venous blood congestion and wetness between the toes.

Diagnosis: Congestive eczema with skin atrophy.

Therapy: Two times daily silica gel diluted with three parts water as a wet compress around the lower legs. Two times each one teaspoon undiluted applied between the toes. Supplementary leg exercises. Total treatment period lasts five weeks.

Pathology: After the second application the itchiness subsides. During further progress itchiness disappears completely and wetness recedes. Only the blood congestion is not satisfactorily improved.

Evaluation: Satisfactory therapeutic efficacy.

Patient 65: K. G., male, 46 years

Clinical Picture: A scraping wound with bruising (hematoma) occurs during therapy for an unrelated condition.

Diagnosis: Skin abrasion with hematoma.

Therapy: Four times daily each one tablespoon silica gel undiluted focally applied to affected skin areas for a total treatment period of 17 days.

Pathology: The pain subsides quickly. The hematoma heals more slowly. After the conclusion of therapy the wound heals broadly.

Evaluation: Good therapeutic efficacy.

Patient 66: A. P., female, 52 years

Clinical Picture: The patient suffers from prematurely aged, loose skin with poor blood flow. Skin easily responds to irritation with reddening.

Diagnosis: Prematurely aged, dried skin.

Therapy: Two times daily one tablespoon silica gel ingested. Evenings: a facial mask with one tablespoon of silica gel diluted with three parts water. This is washed off after 20 minutes. Total treatment period extends over three weeks.

Pathology: As the blood flow through the skin improves only slightly, therapy is stopped early.
Evaluation: Moderate therapeutic efficacy

Patient 67: R. Z., female, 55 years
Clinical Picture: The patient suffers from itchy, taut, often recurring lip blisters.
Diagnosis: Recurring herpes simplex labialis.
Therapy: Four times daily silica gel undiluted focally dabbed on the blisters for a total treatment period of two months.
Pathology: The blisters heal in five days. As the patient breaks off therapy after that, a relapse occurs that cannot be totally healed.
Evaluation: Satisfactory therapeutic efficacy.

Patient 68: B. S., female, 67 years
Clinical Picture: The patient suffers from chronic skin inflammation with reddening mainly in the face.
Diagnosis: Chronic dermatitis.
Therapy: Four times daily one teaspoon silica gel diluted with three parts water focally applied to affected skin areas for a treatment period of 1.5 months.
Pathology: Pain and itchiness subside noticeably after 10 days. Further improvement can be achieved although a complete cure cannot be achieved.
Evaluation: Moderate therapeutic efficacy.

Patient 69: W. F., male, 48 years
Clinical Picture: The patient suffers from skin blemishes. Formerly he had strong acne vulgaris.
Diagnosis: Unclean, oily skin.
Therapy: Two times daily one tablespoon silica gel ingested. At night a facial mask with one tablespoon undiluted silica gel for a half hour. Total treatment period lasts 1.85 months.

Pathology: The skin impurities vanish slowly. The sebaceous secretion normalizes. After the conclusion of therapy there are fewer impurities. The skin has lost most of its excessive oily shine.

Evaluation: Satisfactory therapeutic efficacy.

Patient 70: P. M., female, 53 years

Clinical Picture: The patient suffers from loose, drooping skin that is badly supplied with blood and has protruding veins.

Diagnosis: Connective tissue weakness, premature aging.

Therapy: One tablespoon silica gel ingested daily. Facial mask with one tablespoon diluted with three parts water for 15 minutes, for a total treatment period of 10 weeks.

Pathology: Already after two weeks the skin appears fresher and blood flow through the skin is increased. These improvements continue so that, after the treatment period, the skin visibly rejuvenates.

Evaluation: Good therapeutic efficacy.

Patient 71: N. D., male, 50 years

Clinical Picture: The patient suffers from strong sweating of the hands, feet and armpits. There is chronic irritation and reddening of these areas.

Diagnosis: Hyperidrosis with localized skin damage.

Therapy: Two to three times daily one tablespoon silica gel, diluted with three parts water, focally applied to affected skin areas for a total treatment period of six weeks.

Pathology: Within a short period sweat formation and reddening clearly abate. At the conclusion of therapy there is only slightly excessive sweating without appreciable skin reddening.

Evaluation: Satisfactory therapeutic efficacy.

Patient 72: T. L., female, 54 years

Clinical Picture: During an unrelated therapy, the patient suffered from a slight burn to her hand.

Diagnosis: First degree burn.

Therapy: Three times daily a small portion of silica gel, diluted with three parts water, focally applied to affected skin areas for a total treatment period of 15 days.

Pathology: Just a few hours after the first application, there is noticeable lessening of burn pain. During the further treatment course, the burn heals without any complications.

Evaluation: Good therapeutic efficacy.

Patient 73: F. I., male, 59 years

Clinical Picture: The patient complains of chronically recurring widespread allergic skin eruptions on back and breast with strong itchiness.

Diagnosis: Chronically recurring skin allergy.

Therapy: Four times daily silica gel diluted with three parts water broadly applied to affected skin areas for a total treatment period of four weeks.

Pathology: Already on the second day the itchiness becomes milder. During the further course of treatment, the reddening recedes. On one occasion the allergy flares up again. After that there is only quickly passing itchiness following the consumption of coffee.

Evaluation: Good therapeutic efficacy.

Practical experience with silica gel gleaned from differing skin, hair and nail ailments clearly recommends silica for external application, supplemented with internal ingestion where required for such diseased anomalies that often relate to connective tissue weakness.

Bone and Joint Diseases

Silica acts like a tug for calcium. It promotes the implanting of calcium mineral into the bones. So it is recommended in cases of bone fractures for the cicatrisation (scarring over) of the fracture. It serves similarly during the active growing phases of childhood and youth. It also should be given for the prevention of bone decalcification, i.e., the prevention of osteoporosis, especially for women 35 years and older.

Silica gel is also recommended in cases of intervertebral disk damage and rheumatism of the joint areas. Rheumatologists prescribe silica gel for elasticity diseases affecting the joints (periarticular elastopathies) since it restores tissue elasticity.

Silica gel furthers the elasticity of the intervertebral disks and tissues that surround the joints. Chiefly, the ability of the cells to bond with water improves. The improved water bonding helps to normalize the functions of the affected tissues.

These effects were not tested in this field study because of the length of time required for such a particular study. The effects are of course empirically known from practical medical experience. A silica gel treatment course of one to two tablespoons of silica gel daily over a period of three to four months (or longer) is required to cause the above-described results.

Chapter Nine

It is possible to think that the origin of biological transmutations could be this "liberation" of energy, under particular conditions, in the colloidal medium of living cells when coenzyme metal is present.

Dr. de Larebeyrette, May 1965

Biological Transmutation - Miracle of 2000 and Beyond

Biological trace element research involving silicon is quickly becoming a focus of modern scientific endeavor. A mid-1996 study[*] done with two groups of calves (one group as placebo on choline only) used a stabilized orthosilicic acid to determine the bioavailability of silicon stabilized by the amine choline ($C_5H_{15}NO_2$) and water.

While absorption and bioavailability of silicon were good (using a colloidal silica supplementation), a significant relationship was found between silicon and calcium serum concentrations following administration of only silica! Also magnesium concentration was marginally affected! Furthermore, effects of silicon supplementation showed on phosphor as well. All of these elements are vital in the formation of bone matrix.

[*] Mario R. Calomme, Dirk A. Vanden Berghe, Department of Pharmaceutical Studies, University of Antwerp (UIA), Belgium: *Supplementation of calves with stabilized orthosilicic acid effect on the Si, Ca, Mg and P concentration in serum and on the collagen concentration in skin and cartilage*, 1996, published in Vol 53, number 2, *Biological Trace Element Research* Journal.

Considering the concentrations of silicon and calcium found in serum and in cartilage, the researchers suggest that silicon is involved not only in extracellular matrix components but also in calcium metabolism. The unexplained increase in magnesium and phosphor, though minor, and therefore dismissed by the researchers as insignificant, except that these elements too, are necessary for bone metabolism, perhaps suggests something entirely different: I wonder if we have here a classical manifestation of Professor Kervran's biological transmutation theory? After all, where did the extra calcium (and magnesium and phosphor) come from?

The inhibitory effect silicic acid has on aluminum, which is found in much drinking water and therefore hard to avoid, has also been insufficiently explained. Does the aluminum become attached to silicon and thereby is made harmless? Or is it perhaps transmuted into silicon?

Endoplasmic Transmutation
Recent scientific reviews give ever more credence to the theories of Professor Louis Kervran that he expounded in his book *Biological Transmutations*. Kervran says that, "Incomprehensible as it seems, there nevertheless is in nature a constant movement from certain biological elements into other life elements." There has long been scientific reluctance to accept his extraordinary theory.

The reluctance is understandable if we consider the laws of chemistry laid down in the 18th century by Lavoisier. He established the conservation of matter under all conditions. Lavoisier claimed that there is no spontaneous creation, that "nothing creates itself, in every operation, or reaction, there is an equal quantity of matter before and after... there is only exchange or modification."

In other words, nothing is lost and nothing is created. Instead, every thing can undergo a *transformation* and become a different thing. Stopping short of *transmutation*, Lavoisier's law of the conservation of matter states that the integrity or existence of an individual elementary atom, for example, a silicon atom, is preserved under all conditions. If it disappears at one point in a chemical reaction, it must reappear at another point. Thus a silicon atom cannot, according to Lavoisier, change into, let's say a calcium atom. This scientific law is still widely accepted. There is however glaring conflict that emerged with the Twentieth century.

Radioactive Transmutation
As is now well known, in nuclear reactions certain elements transmute into pure energy. They are no longer matter at all. The atomic age showed that in physical reactions at least matter is not always preserved. Matter can turn into pure energy through spontaneous nuclear disintegration. This is a natural process called radioactivity and was discovered but yet more French scientists, the Curies.

Scientists have attempted at least to explain radioactive transmutation of matter by applying to it Albert Einstein's theory of relativity. With the formula $E = mc2$, Einstein proved mathematically that at the velocity of light (c), energy (E) is equal to mass (m). Einstein's theory had never been studied from the biological viewpoint. Because of variances in the theoretical law of the conservation of mass and energy, science could not explain fully just how biological transmutation may occur.

Dr. Kervran, on the 'a priori' evidence before him, pointed out that biological transmutation exists. He further inferred that it affects every phase of our living things. By change we create life, and life, Kervran reasoned, does not fall within the limitations set by Einsteinian physics. The study of the continuous transmutational life processes in vivo, that is, in the living body, was something more than could be explained by biology, physics or chemistry.

Need Calcium? Take Silica!

The problem of biological transmutation first occurred to Kervran when he was still a boy. He grew up in an area full of slate and granite, rock composed of quartz, feldspar, and mica, but absolutely void of limestone, a rock composed of calcium carbonate. His parents kept chickens that never receive` any limestone, nor was their diet in any way supplemented with limestone. Yet every day during the egg-laying season the chickens laid eggs with calcareous shells.

Young Kervran observed that the chickens were incessantly scratching for mica strewn around the yard. Mica, with feldspar and quartz, contains silica. Why did those chickens search for mica when they need calcium? He watched his mother open the gizzards of slaughtered chickens. They contained grains of sand, but never any mica. What had happened to the mica? How did the calcium get into the eggshell in an area lacking calcium?

The older Kervran learned that already in 1822 the British scientist William Prout had made a systematic comparative study of the amounts of calcium in chicken eggs and the chickens hatched from them. To his bewilderment Prout found that the newly born baby chick contained four times more calcium than there was in the egg. Where did the extra calcium originate? He speculated that there was an unknown element that could transmute into calcium, but he never proved it. The calcium in the eggshell was still intact and, in any event, no calcium could cross the embryonic membrane separating the chicken from the eggshell.

Simultaneously in Germany, another researcher, Vogel, found more sulfur in the sprouts of watercress he was studying, than were present in seeds grown only in pure, distilled water. He concluded from this discrepancy that sulfur could not be a "simple element." He was wrong, of course because sulfur is an element, but where did the extra sulfur come from?

Around 1870, researchers Rothamsted, Lawes and Gilbert found that plants abstracted more magnesium from the soil than it contained. In his professional capacity, Kervran kept coming across ever more unexplained phenomena, similar in nature to the mysterious apparent calcium creation in the shells of chicken eggs and in baby chicks. He also found the same calcium inconsistencies in reptilian eggs. The chicken and egg enigma that had puzzled Prout was eventually explained by researcher Charnot. He found that the membrane that separates the egg from the eggshell contains silica. For 100 g of membrane, there are 154.79 mg of silica (SiO_2) in the inner leaf and 464.80 mg of silica in the outer leaf.

Finally in 1959, Kervran tackled the problem of explaining the biological transmutation of silica into calcium. He had noticed that siliceous stone in sculptures deteriorates over time. Gypsum or carbonate of lime forms, which ultimately disintegrates. Considering his study of ion exchange and many other observations, Kervran assumed that biological transmutations of weak catalyzed energy take place in living organisms. With the assistance of enzymes they can transmute ions of one element into ions of another element and can literally "melt" these ions to form new ions. "In the same way," Kervran concludes, "calcium can result from the fusion of:

      1 ion Mg(magnesium) (=24) + 1 ion O(oxygen) (=16)
or: 2 ions C(carbon) (=12x2) + 1 ion O(oxygen) (=16)
or: 1 ion C(carbon) (=12) + 1 ion Si(silicon) (=28)."

In other words, according to Kervran, both magnesium and silica can be principal sources of calcium in the human body. This astounding hypothesis does explain some well-documented observations, most importantly:

1.   the recalcifying action of silica in growth and in tuberculosis cases.

2.   the human body can excrete more calcium than it receives, the extra calcium coming mainly from magnesium ions.

3.   the calcification of atheroma: "calcium deposits itself when silica diminishes, as though a calcium-silicon balance were a normal metabolic condition"—the transformation of silicon and calcium explains the noted increase in calcium.

Before considering Kervran's conclusions, let us take a closer look at the various interactions of which silica is obviously capable in living tissue.

Biological Metamorphosis
In living bodies, silicon changes to calcium according to this formula: 14 silicon atoms plus 6 carbon atoms create 20 calcium atoms. Kervran points to the examples of the earthworms and microorganisms known as streptomyces that transmute silica into calcium. Two other researchers, Berthelot and Andre, described the biological interdependence of silica and phosphorus and how silica promotes the assimilation of phosphorus. Phosphorus tissue easily retains silica so that one can find silica in the phosphorus-rich brain tissue. It follows that when phosphorus therapy or supplementation is prescribed, simultaneous supplementary silica therapy should be considered. Not surprisingly, both silica and phosphorus are of special significance in the treatment

of many nervous disorders, most famously Alzheimer's disease. They are also helpful in the relief of asthenia, a debilitating body weakness.

Charnot could "reattach" silica to the random migrations of calcium and phosphorus in horses. Silica diminished in all the following body functions and organs: in bile, the adrenal, cartilage, teeth, muscles, nails, skin, hair, lungs, spleen and blood. In the teeth and bones, normally important reserves of silica and calcium, all traces of silica vanished. Nerve tissues like the brain, cerebellum and marrow, rich in phosphorus, registered a silica increase.

It seems that all problems in calcium metabolism are caused by decalcification (as in tuberculosis) or by hypercalcification (as in bone). Calcium migrations seem to provoke an exaggerated consumption of body silica, while the storage of body silica in the nervous tissue suggests two possible reasons:

1)   the organism during the reorganization of its silica, stores it in phosphor-rich tissues because they are best suited to contain it.

2)   a substitution for silica or phosphorus has formed in the presence of an excess of circulating silica. Two other researchers, Hall and Morisson, have shown that silica can replace phosphates.

At this point, Kervran conducted research to confirm the bond between calcium, potassium and magnesium. To prove transmutation of potassium to calcium, he put hens into a chicken run and left them without access to lime. After some days they had used all their calcium reserves and laid soft-shelled eggs. On that day they were given pure mica. The hens, controlled from birth, had never seen mica, but fell upon it with relish. The following day the eggs had normal shells! Kervran concluded that in this case the transmuted calcium came from potassium.

Sodium is very similar to potassium. Kervran claims that in human beings potassium can transmute from sodium. However, sodium is associated with several ailments, notably high blood pressure in which sodium intake might have to be reduced. Therefore, to combat potassium deficiency, he suggests absorbable magnesium, or, even better, silica!

Biological Balance

Kervran found imbalances of the elements that could not be reconciled with the existing law of the conservation of matter. The sciences of biology (life study) and chemistry (matter study) had to merge into the separate, new science of biochemistry. The new science could better explain the behavior of chemicals inside living matter. While many interactions of living matter are produced by traceable chemical reactions, in biochemistry the unperceived phenomenon of transmutation takes place.

Kervran states that, "The chemistry of the living organism is essentially different from the chemistry in the lab." Chemists require very high temperatures and great pressures to create reactions. The same reactions occur inside living matter at much lower temperatures and less pressure. The human organism, for instance, makes this possible through living enzymes that catalyze endless biological reactions. The elements involved in these transmutations are all highly unstable - but so is life!

Chemistry and nuclear physics study dead matter "in vitro." This type of analysis, Kervran reasons, can neither understand nor explain biological transmutation - so it denies its existence. They base their reluctance on findings that are unrelated to life and living functions. "Physicists do not deny the presence of an energy that maintains life, but for them this energy comes from what the organism takes in from its surrounding outside medium. They do not realize the great flaw in their argument," says Kervran.

The principle of entropy, Kervran holds, has never been applicable to biology. "It was formed only for closed systems having no exchange with the outside; therefore the ideas of entropy and negentropy (negative entropy) have no significance when there is an exchange with the outside medium." Questioning the applicability of entropy to the "human system," Kervran prompts, "Who is to say in which present day branch of physics mental energy,' the strength of will or character, should be placed?"

The most eminent physicist of our time, was also one of the wisest. In his research Einstein allowed for scientific doubt, expansion of existing scientific ideas, and an overriding God! However, to remain scientific, let me repeat that Professor Kervran's biological transmutation regarding the workings of silica is a theory. Like all theories, it must be questioned repeatedly for verification.

Today I find it somewhat easier to accept biological transmutation. Since first writing about Kervran, I have been and am still studying electromagnetic effects on living tissue. Electromagnetic frequencies, I now know, cause physical and chemical changes merely by their vibrations. Silica, a semiconductor of electrical energy in crystal form also creates vibration energy. Perhaps one day soon we will find that there is something that Albert Einstein was looking for in the last days of his life; a unified field theory!

Chapter Ten

"O blessed health! thou art above all gold and treasure, the poor man's riches, the rich man's bliss."

Robert Burton,
The Anatomy of Melancholy, 1621

Gathering Great Gel Gems

Bathing in Kieselsäure Balsam

Does your skin suffer from injuries, open sores, eczemas, sunburn or other problems? Then soaking in a tub of warm water permeated with silica gel can become a cruise that slowly takes your skin to the wanted destinations of restored health and beauty. Can you add silica gel safely to your bath water? In Germany "Kieselsäurebäder," (Kieselsäure is the German for silicic acid, i.e., silica gel) are taken at spas. In 1938 researcher Lambert reported that minerals, including silica, produce displacement of electrolytes in the skin while bathing in them. In the 1950s orthodox medicine still laughed at bathing in mineral waters and in the USA such treatments were even prohibited by the FDA.

Dr. Paavo Airola, America's number one nutritionist during the 1980s, provides great insight into the skin's absorptive powers. His experiments call into question the generally held scientific view that nutrient substances, including silica gel, cannot penetrate healthy skin. In startling human experiments, he showed that the rubbing of garlic on the

159

soles of the feet causes the garlic to enter the bloodstream. This was witnessed because shortly after this procedure, people, who did not regularly eat garlic, could taste the garlic on their tongues! You may wish to repeat this experiment for yourself at home.

A silica gel dispersion applied externally can have a tonic effect not just on damaged skin but also on overall health. Given silica's cancer-fighting ability, it may deter the formation of cancerous moles. This is of increasing concern in a world where ultraviolet radiation from the sun is greatly increased due to the destruction of the ozone layer. I am suggesting that silica gel applied externally could have a positive effect on the basal epidermis layers. This would certainly help to keep melanocytes, the cells that give rise to tanning, from becoming deadly by mutating into the most dangerous form of skin cancer: melanoma. This is, however, not confirmed by research.

However, silica is well-known to have a positive tonic effect on blood vessels. Burst capillary vessels, so-called spider veins, can form on the skin of susceptible individuals. Regular bathing in silica gel may prevent their formation or diminish those formed. This also goes for so-called liver or age spots that are caused by excessive exposure to ultraviolet radiation.

If a kind of osmosis occurs, i.e., the passage of the silica solvent through the skin, then bathing in silica gel would also positively influence the deeper connective tissues, the dermis and subcutaneous tissue. This would be wonderful news, because the lower vascular layers of the dermis consist mainly of collagen, which is intimately connected to silica. The dermis is rich in blood vessels and sensory nerves. The collagen layers support and strengthen the epidermis. This could also affect hair growth by stimulating the hair roots directly. I will put this to the test on myself over the next few years.

I must inform you that the scientists at the silica gel lab in Germany state that even their finely dispersed colloidal silica gel cannot penetrate unbroken skin. But listen to the advice of Dr. Rudolf Fritz Weiss, M.D. In his well-respected book *Herbal Medicine* (1988), Weiss specifically advocates the therapeutic use of silica baths for hand, foot and body. Weiss ascribes a specific action to skin metabolism, subcutaneous cell tissue, and also ligaments and tendons. This indicates silica bathing to be helpful in cases of ankle fractures or sprains, as well as all symptoms due to dropped arches and flat feet. He goes on to cite silica bathing for rheumatic and neuralgic conditions, chronic eczema and neurodermatitic conditions. Silica baths are also indicated for local peripheral vascular disorders, chilblains and post-thrombotic swelling.

If that is not convincing, Maria Treben, the world-famous herbalist from Austria, recommends bathing in horsetail because of its high silica content. Colloidal silica gel, because of its instant dispersion in water and its facilitated absorption, may be better suited for bathing use than a horsetail extract or concoction. This definitely holds true for injured skin. In any event, if you care to try it out in your own bathtub, it is certainly very simple to prepare a silica gel bath. All you need to do is add a reasonable amount of silica gel to warm bath water.

Keep in mind though that external applications should be fortified with internal supplementation. The good news is that you never need to worry about overusing colloidal silica gel. It is quite non-poisonous. If fact, according to researcher Carlisle, there is no danger of overdosing with silica up to fairly well-defined limits.

Desiccant Silica Gel – Or What's in a Name?

For dietary purposes, silica gel must be clearly distinguished from any of the dry industrial silica gels that are manufactured as an agent for filtering, dehumidifying and dehydrating. Never confuse colloidal mineral silica gel with other silica or silica gel products, and especially not with industrial silica gel products. I was reminded of this the other day when a new baby grand piano arrived at our neighbor's house.

I was invited for the unpacking ceremony and privileged to listen to the first precious tune. Except that, while everyone else was raptly following the player's fingers dancing over the shiny new keyboard, I glanced down and saw something that had fallen on the rug. I picked it up, and looked at it. Was I ever startled out of musical reveries when I read this message: "Throw Away – Desiccant Silica Gel – Do Not Eat – Throw Away." Desiccant silica gels are specifically formulated to adsorb water, whereas dietary silica gel is silica suspended in water.

Silica Gel Forecast

Silica research is ongoing, including my own investigative research of silica gel. Currently under investigation in California is the role silicon plays with other elements like aluminum and molybdenum. As indicated in the beginning, silica's comparative absorption rate in human beings is under study. There is every indication that the future outlook for silica gel therapy is very promising.

To forecast your own silica needs, measuring the amount of silicon currently traceable in your body is a good beginning. The easiest way of determining body silicon content is through a careful hair analysis. A hair analysis is like shooting a time-exposure photo over a period of several weeks or months or even years, depending on the length of your hair.

The trace elements in your system are eventually deposited into your hair shafts. As indicated earlier, so-called "normal" values for hair silicon are in excess of 20 ppm. Lower counts might indicate a silica gel deficiency, but in the very least, should be followed with a connective tissue or blood analysis before commencing therapy.

The only hair analysis report of trace elements that includes a reading for silicon, and that I know of, is available through the Alive Academy of Nutrition. You can reach the Academy by telephoning (604) 435-1919, faxing (604) 435-4888, or sending your written request to Box 80055, Burnaby, BC V5H 3X1. The results of your hair analysis will offer you vital clues for silica gel supplementation. You will find that a lot of labs are not equipped to check for silicon content because of using glass vials in analysis. So, whatever you decide, make sure you obtain an accurate report. If necessary, ask the performing lab how they measure for silicon. If you want to find out more details about hair analysis, you may want to read the book *Trace Elements, Hair Analysis and Nutrition* by Richard A. Passwater, Ph.D. and Elmer M. Cranton, M.D.

Do I supplement with silica? You bet! I supplement with different silica sources similar to my practice of supplementing with both vitamin A and provitamin A or carotene. I also supplement with various sources of other trace elements, such as zinc. In addition, I apply colloidal silica gel externally.

It took uncounted steps to bring life on earth to its present stage of higher development. Today's humanity has matured to the role of caretaker. We are no longer mere subjects of nature's forces of evolution. Our new task is unpolluting our world or risk being thrown out again from the earthly Garden of Eden by the flaming sword of pollution, this time for good.

Our own body is the best place to start and will impact on our environment. As within, so without! By cleansing our bodies, we are taking an active part in reducing environmental pollution. As all of the earth's crust is siliceous, except for carbonate and phosphate rocks, silica, in such tremendous abundance, will play an increasingly crucial role in the future health of the world and of mankind.

"Live long and prosper!"[30]

Endnotes

1. Edith Muriel Carlisle, School of Public Health, University of California (UCLA), Los Angeles, CA, USA, Chapter 7, "Silicon" in *Trace Elements in Human and Animal Nutrition,* Vol. 2, 1986, Academic Press, Inc.

2. Edith Muriel Carlisle, Ph.D., School of Public Health, University of California (UCLA), Los Angeles, CA "Silicon" in *Trace Elements in Human and Animal Nutrition,* Vol. 2, 1986, Academic Press, Inc.

3. See Volume I, *Silica – The Forgotten Nutrient*, Chapter 3, p. 11.

4. According to Ernst A. Hauser, Ph.D., Sc.D., Professor of Colloid Science, Massachusetts Institute of Technology, in his book *Silica Science* on page 175, "Pharmaceutical Applications."

5. See Volume I, *Silica – The Forgotten Nutrient* for a detailed explanation of horsetail-derived silica.

6. According to Hauschka (1950).

7. As per researcher Fuhrmann (1972).

8. Established according to A. H. Schweigart (1962).

9. According to Flamm-Kroeber-Seel.

10. According to Robert and Gonnermann.

11. *Über die Toxizitätsprüfung von Silicea-Balsam,* Pharmakologisch-Analytisches Institut, D-8191 Gelting, Germany: 2 Jan. 1980: Report #912131.

12. By D. Werner in 1968.

13. According to researcher B. Kober.

14. Sclerosol with Dr. Kobbe.

15. According to Gohr and Scholl (Dr. Kobbe: sclerosol).

16. According to research by M. H. Fischer.
17. Confirmed by Saller.
18. According to Robin and More (1909).
19. According to Robin.
20. Confirmed by Saller.
21. This theory has been confirmed through successful application for carcinomas and sarcomas as reported in the work of Villanova and Caballis, Hesse, Wiesinger, Poras, Kranfelder, Dahrowolsky (see B. Kober 1955). Stiegele (see Metzger, p. 654) reports a case of intestinal cancer that healed with silica.
22. As shown by the UCLA studies under Prof. Dr. Carlisle.
23. As in rat experiments by C. Waentz and proven also in humans.
24. Nancy Appleton, Ph.D., *Healthy Bones: What You Should Know About Osteoporosis.* Avery Publishing Group, Garden City Park, NY, 1991.
25. Anderson, Robert A., M.D., *Wellness Medicine.* Keats Publishing Inc., New Canaan,CT, 1990.
26. Mowrey, Daniel B., Ph.D., *Vegetable Sources of Silicon.* In press, 1991.
27. By Group' Besanez.
28. According to researcher Herman Hädeler. His view is confirmed by researcher Galler.
29. The study results (written in German) are available for health professionals and organizations for a small user fee. English translations can be obtained for a negotiable fee. Only serious inquiries should be addressed to the author directly at: 9566 Willowleaf Place, Burnaby, BC, V5A 4A5, Canada.
30. This last wish is Dr. Zoltan Rona's suppressed message for all you science fiction fans. In reference to the movie "Star Trek," Dr. Rona suggested, "as someone well-nourished with silica from the 24th century once said, "Live long and prosper." He left it out because it was felt that it might be misunderstood. I just had to acknowledge this in an endnote at least.

Bibliography

Ahrens, L.H. et al. eds. 1959. *Physics and chemistry of the earth.* Vol. 3.

Anderson, R.A. M.D. 1990. *Wellness medicine.* New Canaan: Keats Publishing Inc.

Antweiler, H. 1955. *Journal for the Society of Experimental Medicine,* 126:353.

Arch. Hyg. 1956. 138:22. Arch. tissue path. Tissue Hyg. 15: 158

Baumeister, M.D., Herne I.W. 1950. The general practitioner's treatment of lung tuberculosis and tuberculotics, pleurisy. Vol. 4, Colloidal silicon in the hands of the general practitioner. Otto & Co.

Berthelot and André, cp. Monceaux 1959.

Birkhofer, L. and Ritter, H. 1958. *Liebig's annals of chemistry.* 612:22

Bloss, F.D. 1971. *Crystal chemistry.*

Breitenstein, see Warning.

Bürger, M. 1958. *Journal of age research.* 10:20.

Butenandt cp. 1958. Manegold, E., General and applied colloid science. Heidelberg.

Charnot, cp. Monceaux.

Clarck, Dr K. *Plant Juices.* (Dr. Schweizer, M.D. Editions, Reutlingen-Pfullingen)

Deer, W.A., et al. 1963. *Rock-forming minerals,* Vol. 4, 2A, 2d ed. 1979.

Dohrowolsky 1955. *The role of silica with lung tuberculosis.* Polish Gazette Lek 7, 29 and see Kober.

Deters, H., cp. Warning.

Domagk. 1965 Nobel prize meeting. Lindau.

Dröre 1950. Personal publication to Otto & Co.

167

Eitel, W., ed. 1965-66. *Silicate science,* 4 vols.

Engel, W. and Holzapfel, L. 1953. *Planta.* 41, 358.

Fischer, M.H. 1951. *The Formation of living substance.* Steinkopff: Darmstadt.

Flamm, Kroeber, and Seel, *Prescription book for medicinal plants.*

Fuhrmann, E. 1927. *The Chemistry of food and luxury.* Berlin: Urban and Schwarzenberg.

Geiger, H. 1963. *Rehabilitation.* 165, 6.

Gohr, H. 1950. *Medical practice.* 11:20.

Group-Besanez, cp. H. Warning 1947.

Graham, T., cp. Monceaux 1959.

Hädeler, Hermann, and Hildesheim, (Undated). Silica: Professional further education. 3:72, 1st year.

Haurowitz, F. 1935. *Journal of physiological chemistry.* 182, 82, 232, 153.

Hauschka, R. 1950. Substance study. Frankfurt :Klostermann.

Hauser, E.A. 1955. *Silicic Science.* Princeton: D. van Nostrand Co. Inc.

Heinen, W. 1965. *Silicon metabolism in microorganisms.* Vol. 7.

Hendler, S.S., M.D. 1990. *The Doctor's vitamin and mineral encyclopedia.* New York: Simon and Schuster.

Hesse 1937. *Advanced Therapy.* Vol. 13.

Hesse, E., *Applied pharmacology.* 101 ff.

Hiepe, F. 1970. *Silica.* Company report of Anton Hübner Co., Kirchhofen.

Holzapfel, L. 1949. *Coll. Journal.* Vols. 115, 137.

Hurlbut, C. and Klein, C. 1977. *Manual of mineralogy.* After J.D. Dana, 19th ed.

Iler, R.K. 1979. *The Chemistry of silica.*

Jäger, R. 1953. *Scientific activity report 63.* Münster.

Joetten and Klosterkötter 1958. *Medicine.* p. 1,075.

Jung, Dr. 1948. *On the history of medicinal soils.* The Pharmacy 6 (3rd year): 278 ff.

Kervran, C.L. 1980. *Biological Transmutations.* Woodstock: Beekman Publishers, Inc.

Kober, B. 1955. *Munich Med.* Weekly 23, 767.

Kobert. On silica containing remedies especially with tuberculosis.

Kochmann, L. and Maier, L. 1930. *Biochemical journal.* 223, 228.

Kohler, K. 1956. *Munich medical weekly.* 23, 767.

Kollath, W. 1947. "Ordering of nutrition." in *Textbook of Hygiene*, 2nd Edition. Leipzig:Hirzl.

Kosaki, T., Ikoda, T., Kotani, Y., Kakagawa, S. and Saka, T. 1958. *Science.* 127, 3307.

Kranfelder. The Significance of silica content in blood of tuberculotics. See Kober 1955.

Kühn 1901. Pflüger's archives. Vol. 67.

Kühn 1917. *Journal of physiological chemistry.* 99:296

Kühn 1921. *German medical weekly.* 38:673

Kühn 1923. *Journal of clinical tuberculosis.* 47:296

Kühn 1949. *Therapeutic weekly.* Vol. 4

Kühn. Silica, its peroral, parenteral, and prebronchial application and effect with internal diseases. *Dental world* p. 497. Lampert. Physical therapy.

Leibold, G. 1984. *Kieselsäure-Urquell des Lebens.* Karlsruhe:V.G.L.-Verlage.

Lindemann, G. Silica from a biochemical and phytotherapeutic view.

Loeper. See Monceaux 1959.

Mahr, H. 1959. Correspondence report to Otto & Co.

Mezger, J. 1950. Inspected homeopathic pharmacology, Ulm Company publication.

Moleschott 1852. Circulation of life. ibid Struve and Brock.

Monceaux, A.H. 1959. "Hospital week of Paris." The hospital no. 690:19, 148

Moninger, W. 1935. Dissertation, Munich Technical College.

Montpellier, cp. Monceaux.

Mowrey, D.B. 1991. Vegetable sources of silicon. In press.

Nauhof, K. H. 1949. Report to Dr. Becker laboratory.

Pasteur, L., cp. Monceaux 1959.

Patzelt, V. 1948. *Histology,* 3rd Edition, Berlin: Urban & Schwarzenberg.

Pearce, C. A. 1972. *Silicon chemistry and applications.* London: The Chemical Society.

Plagniol, cp. Monceaux 1959.

Poras, cp. Kober 1955.

Rabat, cp. Monceaux

Robin, cf. Reiff 1932. Collected proof of accuracy of mineral salt therapy, and cf. Monceaux 1959.

Rona, Z.P. 1991. *The Joy of Health,* 68. Article/letter to the author re Silica vs. Calcium citrate.

Rondoni, P. 1937. *Journal of cancer research.* 47:59. Rondoni, P. Swiss medical weekly 78/18:419.

Rondoni, P. 1949. Cancer physician 7/8:251. Rößle and Kahle, cf. Reiff.

Scholl, O. and Letter, K. 1959. *Munich medical weekly* 101/50, 2321.

Schomerus. Biodynamic economic methods in fruit and garden construction.

Schulz, H. 1920. "Addresses on the effect and application of inorganic pharmaceuticals." In Inorganic pharmaceuticals, 4th Edition. Leipzig:Thieme.

Schweigart, H.A. 1962. Vital material table. Dachau: Zauer Editions.

Seeger, P.G., M.D. 1937. Archives of experiential cell research 20:280. Berlin:Falkensee.

Seeger, P.G., M.D. 1938. ibid. 21:306, 22:332.

Seeger, P.G., M.D. 1939. *Journal of microbiotic anatomical research.* 48:181, 631, 639, 53, 65;

Seeger, P.G., M.D. 1951. *Journal of cancer research.* 57:387.

Seeger, P.G., M.D. 1970. The vital significance of silica; Natural medicine practice Vols. 7, 8, 1973; Silicon - the elixir of life; Folk medical science, 1972. Complete bibliography of Ferenczi-Seeger-Trüb, Red Beet Book. Haug Editions.

Stiegele, cf. 1950. Mezger, 554.

Susman, R.B. 1965. The Phases of Silica.

Unna, C.P. 1917. *Dermatological weekly.* 64.

Villanova and Cabalis 1935. Bulletin of the academy of medicine. Paris II.

Waentz, C., cf. Lindemann.

Wagner 1940. The Importance of silica in the growth of some cultivated plants. *Phytopathological journal* 7:5.

Warning, H. 1947. The Treatment of inflammations with silica. Königstein: Königstein Technical College; Pleinböhl: Pleinböhl Teacher's College.

Werner, D. 1981. Botanical society report. 9:425.

Willheim, R. and Stern, K. 1936. The paths and results of chemical cancer research. Vienna: Aesculap Editions.

Wiesinger 1935. Tuberculosis 15.

Index

A

abscesses, 70, 92-93, 96-97, 119
absorption, 31, 75, 85, 89-90, 96, 149, 161-162
adrenal, 155
adsorbent, 32, 34
aerosol, 21
age spots, 160
AIDS, 67, 75-77
albumen, 25, 33
albuminoid, 30
albumins, 49-50
alkaline silicates, 27
allergies, 142
alum, 54
aluminosilicates, 13
aluminum, 13-14, 150, 162
Alzheimer's, 13-14, 155
amenorrhea, 82
amino acids, 33, 49-50
amphoteric, 49
anabolic, 8
angina, 96
anhydride, 29
anti-aging, 44, 48
anti-degenerative, 44
anti-inflammatory, 7, 32, 67-68, 118, 128, 132, 138, 142
antioxidants, 37
aorta, 7
aquifer, 58-59, 61-62
arterial sclerosis, 119

arterial walls, 106, 120
arteries, 7, 74, 119-120
arteriosclerosis, 6, 46, 73-75, 97, 101, 103-104, 119-127
asthenia, 155
atheroma, 154
atherosclerosis, 6, 73-74
atomic number, 10

B

basalt, 58
bed sores, 92
bile, 155
bioavailability, 10, 75, 90, 149
biocatalyst, 42
biochemistry, 17, 50, 86, 156, 172
biological transmutation, 14-15, 149-153, 155, 157
biosensors, 9
blood, 7, 23, 39-40, 46, 49-50, 71, 74-75, 81, 89-90, 99, 119-125, 142-146,
    155-156, 160, 163, 169
blood pressure, 46, 50, 74-75, 119-122, 124-125, 156
blood silica, 46, 90
boils, 92, 119
bone density, 79-80, 82
bone formation, 73, 80, 83-85, 87
bone loss, 80
bone matrix, 83-84, 150
bone pain, 81
bone resorption, 80-81
bone thinning, 79-83, 85-87
bones, 44, 63, 68, 79, 82-86, 95, 148, 155, 166
brain, 14-15, 39-40, 155
brittle nails, 43, 94, 108, 142-143
bronchial catarrh, 101, 103-104, 127-131, 135
bronchitis, 67, 101, 103-104, 127-131, 135
buzzing, 74, 122, 124

C

calcification, 74, 85, 154
calcitonin, 81, 85
calcium, 15, 47, 59-60, 75, 80-86, 95, 138, 148-156
calcium carbonate, 152
calcium phosphate, 47
callouses, 93
carbon, 9-11, 33, 44, 154

D

diathesis, 46, 101, 104, 111, 113
diatom, 34-35, 42
diatomaceous earth, 34
diatomite, 34
dielectric, 9
diuresis, 118
dizziness, 74-75
duodenal ulcer, 69-70
dysopia, 125
dyspepsia, 68

E

eczema, 92, 96-97, 144, 161
edema, 49
elasticity, 7, 16, 49, 66, 91, 93, 106, 127, 148
elastin, 105
electromagnetic, 157
electrorheological, 9
embryonic, 41, 49, 106, 153
empirical, 2, 5, 99
enteritis, 68
entropy, 157
epidermis, 35-36, 160
esters,50
estrogen,80

F

fat metabolism, 35
fatty acid synthesis, 42
feldspar, 13, 152
filtration, 20, 62
flat feet, 161
flatulence, 68, 70, 101, 104, 114-115, 117
fluoridated, 81
fractures, 81, 83, 85, 95, 148, 161
frostbite, 92, 97
furuncles, 69, 93, 97-98, 119

G

gastritis, 69-70, 95, 97, 115
gastroenteritis, 101, 103, 116
gelatine, 26
gelatinous, 3, 28, 34

H

I, J, K

L

M

T

U

V – Z

Recommended Reading

The titles listed below can be purchased or ordered at your local health food store or specialty book store. If unavailable, copies may be ordered directly from the publisher.

Health from God's Garden – Herbal Remedies for Glowing health and Well-Being, Maria Treben, Healing Arts Press, Rochester, Vermont, 1988, 128 pp softcover

Health through God's Pharmacy – Advice and Experiences with Medicinal Herbs, Maria Treben, Wilhelm Ennsthaler Publisher, Austria, 1980, 88 pp softcover

Herbal Medicine, Rudolf Fritz Weiss, Beaconsfield Publishers, Beaconsfield, England, 1988, 362 pp softcover

Trace Elements, Hair Analysis and Nutrition, Richard A. Passwater, Ph.D. and Elmer M. Cranton, M.D., Keats Publishing, Inc., New Canaan, CT, 1983, 385 pp softcover

Return to the Joy of Health – Natural Medicine and Alternative Treatments for All Your Health Complaints, Zoltan P. Rona, MD MSc, Alive Books, Vancouver, BC, 1995 408 pp softcover

Useful Addresses

Alive Academy of Nutrition
7436 Fraser Park Drive
Burnaby BC V5J 5B9
604-435-1919
Fax: 604-435-4888

**Canadian Holistic Medical
Association (A Division of the
Orthomolecular Medical Centre)**
42 Redpath Avenue
Toronto ON M5N 1A8
416-485-3071
Fax: 416-485-3076

**Health Action Network Society
(H.A.N.S.)**
#202 - 5262 Rumble Street
Burnaby BC V5J 2B6
604-435-0512
Fax: 604-435-1561

Safe Water Foundation
6439 Taggart Road
Delaware OH 43015
614-548-5340
John Jamianis, Ph.D.
(biochemistry) Author of
Fluoride – The Aging Factor

Well Mind Association
4649 Sunnyside Avenue North
Seattle WA 98103
206-547-6167

**NatureWorks (Distributed by
Abkit, Inc)**
207 East 94th Street 2nd floor
New York NY 10128
212-860-8358
Fax: 212-860-8323

Purity Life Health Products Ltd
6 Commerce Crescent
Acton ON L7J 2X3
519-853-3511
Fax: 519-853-4660

or

2975 Lake City Way
Burnaby BC V5A 2Z6
604-421-8931
Fax: 416-748-1555

Naka Sales Ltd
53 Queenplate Drive Unit 3
Etobicoke ON M9W 6P1
416-748-3073
Fax: 416-748-1555

Anton Hübner GmbH & Co
Postfach 49 Schloßstraße 11 – 17
D-7801 Ehrenkirchen 1
Germany
011-49-07-633-801-0
Fax: 011-49-07-633-801-48

About the Author

Klaus Kaufmann is mainly self-taught. Historical events of World War II and the turmoil following denied him the privilege of completing university. Yet his thirst for knowledge remained unquenchable. Klaus has been studying natural healing properties for many years. His search for a more natural lifestyle took him all over the globe. Following a photo safari to Africa, he decided to live in Southern Africa for some years. There he obtained first hand knowledge of healing flora, such as the Fever Tree, the bark of which is chewed by the natives to prevent malaria. He then took his wife to the equatorial reaches, spending a year on a teaching permit in Kuala Lumpur, Malaysia. During 1977, the Kaufmanns moved to White Rock, BC to participate actively in miniature horse breeding. Klaus had started the first such horse farm in Canada several years earlier with friends.

In the years that followed, his interest in writing blossomed alongside his growing interest in all matters related to health. Following the study of English literature and creative writing at university, his professor appointed Klaus editor of CONTACT, a Canadian Writers Guild publication. Under his editorship, the publication expanded from a simple newsletter to a magazine. When Klaus left, the publication was popular in book shops and read at universities across Canada and in England. A live performance in Toronto, "Jazz and Poetry" selected Klaus' poetry for a public reading. Before being published under his own name, Klaus worked as a ghost writer.

His enormously popular bestseller, *Silica – The Forgotten Nutrient,* was quickly followed by *The Joy of Juice Fasting,* which made the bestseller list, and *Eliminating Poison in Your Mouth*. Most recently Klaus has been writing books for the "Rediscovered series" by Alive Books. The first smash hit *Kombucha Rediscovered!* was followed by *Kefir Rediscovered!* (March 1997). Klaus and his wife Gabrielle live at the foot of Burnaby Mountain in British Columbia.

Other Titles by Alive Books

The All-in-One Guide to Herbs, Vitamins & Minerals
The quick and easy reference for everything you need to know.
Victoria Hogan, 64pp softcover

Allergies: Disease in Disguise
How to heal your allergic condition permanently and naturally.
Carolee Bateson-Koch DC ND, 224 pp softcover

The Breuss Cancer Cure
Advice for prevention and natural treatment of cancer, leukemia and other seemingly incurable diseases.
Rudolf Breuss (translated from German), 112pp softcover

Devil's Claw Root and Other Natural Remedies for Arthritis
A herbal remedy that has helped free thousands of arthritis sufferers from crippling pain.
Rachel Carston (Revised by Klaus Kaufmann), 128 pp softcover

Diet for All Reasons
Nutrition guide and recipe collection.
Paulette Eisen, 176 pp softcover

Eliminating Poison in Your Mouth
Overcoming mercury amalgam toxicity.
Klaus Kaufmann, 44 pp softcover

Fats That Heal Fats That Kill
The complete guide to fats, oils, cholesterol and human health.
Udo Erasmus, 480 pp softcover

For the Love of Food
The complete natural foods cookbook.
J. M. Martin, 484 pp hardcover

Healing with Herbal Juices
A practical guide to herbal juice therapy: nature's preventative medicine
Siegfried Gursche, 256 pp softcover

Kombucha Rediscovered!
A guide to the medicinal benefits of an ancient healing tea.
Klaus Kaufmann, 96 pp softcover

Living with Green Power
A gourmet collection of raw food recipes.
Elysa Markowitz, 176 pp hardcover

Return to the Joy of Health
Natural medicine and alternative treatments for all your health complaints.
Dr. Zoltan Rona, 408 pp softcover

Silica - The Forgotten Nutrient
A guide to the vital role of organic vegetal silica in nutrition, health, longevity and medicine.
Klaus Kaufmann, 128 pp softcover

All books are available at your local health food store or from **Alive Books**,
PO Box 80055, Burnaby BC V5H 3X1